Vulnerable Children in the United States

Editors

ARTURO BRITO
STEVEN KAIRYS

PEDIATRIC CLINICS
OF NORTH AMERICA

www.pediatric.theclinics.com

Consulting Editor
BONITA F. STANTON

April 2020 • Volume 67 • Number 2

ELSEVIER

1600 John F. Kennedy Boulevard • Suite 1800 • Philadelphia, Pennsylvania, 19103-2899

http://www.theclinics.com

THE PEDIATRIC CLINICS OF NORTH AMERICA Volume 67, Number 2
April 2020 ISSN 0031-3955, ISBN-13: 978-0-323-73352-6

Editor: Kerry Holland
Developmental Editor: Casey Potter

The Pediatric Clinics of North America (ISSN 0031-3955) is published bimonthly by Elsevier Inc., 360 Park Avenue South, New York, NY 10010-1710. Months of issue are February, April, June, August, October, and December. Periodicals postage paid at New York, NY and additional mailing offices. Subscription prices are $240.00 per year (US individuals), $695.00 per year (US institutions), $315.00 per year (Canadian individuals), $924.00 per year (Canadian institutions), $362.00 per year (international individuals), $924.00 per year (international institutions), $100.00 per year (US students and residents), $100.00 per year (Canadian students and residents), and $165.00 per year (international residents and students). To receive students/resident rare, orders must be accompanied by name of affiliated institution, date of term, and the signature of program/residency coordinator on institution letterhead. Orders will be billed at individual rate until proof of status is received. Foreign air speed delivery is included in all *Clinics* subscription prices. All prices are subject to change without notice. **POSTMASTER:** Send address changes to *The Pediatric Clinics of North America*, Elsevier Health Sciences Division, Subscription Customer Service, 3251 Riverport Lane, Maryland Heights, MO 63043. **Customer Service: 1-800-654-2452 (US and Canada). From outside of the US and Canada: 1-314-447-8871. Fax: 1-314-447-8029. For print support, E-mail: JournalsCustomerService-usa@elsevier.com. For online support, E-mail: JournalsOnlineSupport-usa@elsevier.com.**

Reprints. For copies of 100 or more, of articles in this publication, please contact the Commercial Reprints Department, Elsevier Inc., 360 Park Avenue South, New York, NY 10010-1710. Tel.: 212-633-3874; Fax: 212-633-3820; E-mail: reprints@elsevier.com.

The Pediatric Clinics of North America is also published in Spanish by McGraw-Hill Inter-americana Editores S.A., Mexico City, Mexico; in Portuguese by Riechmann and Affonso Editores, Rua Comandante Coelho 1085, CEP 21250, Rio de Janeiro, Brazil; and in Greek by Althayia SA, Athens, Greece.

The Pediatric Clinics of North America is covered in *MEDLINE/PubMed (Index Medicus), Excerpta Medica, Current Contents, Current Contents/Clinical Medicine, Science Citation Index, ASCA, ISI/BIOMED,* and *BIOSIS*.

PROGRAM OBJECTIVE

The goal of the *Pediatric Clinics of North America* is to keep practicing physicians and residents up to date with current clinical practice in pediatrics by providing timely articles reviewing the state-of-the-art in patient care.

TARGET AUDIENCE

All practicing pediatricians, physicians and healthcare professionals who provide patient care to pediatric patients.

LEARNING OBJECTIVES

Upon completion of this activity, participants will be able to:

1. Review the epidemiology, clinical features, treatment options and barriers to treatment for the pediatric population experiencing abuse and select adverse childhood experiences
2. Discuss evidence-based care for the pediatric population experiencing abuse and select adverse childhood experiences
3. Recognize the clinical presentation, diagnosis and recommended best practices to manage child abuse and select adverse childhood experiences

ACCREDITATIONS

Physician Credit

The Elsevier Office of Continuing Medical Education (EOCME) is accredited by the Accreditation Council for Continuing Medical Education (ACCME) to provide continuing medical education for physicians.

The EOCME designates this journal-based activity for a maximum of 13 *AMA PRA Category 1 Credit*(s)™. Physicians should claim only the credit commensurate with the extent of their participation in the activity.

All other healthcare professionals requesting continuing education credit for this this journal-based activity will be issued a certificate of participation.

ABP Maintenance of Certification Credit

Successful completion of this CME activity, which includes participation in the activity and individual assessment of and feedback to the learner, enables the learner to earn up to 13 MOC points in the American Board of Pediatrics' (ABP) Maintenance of Certification (MOC) program. It is the CME activity provider's responsibility to submit learner completion information to ACCME for the purpose of granting ABP MOC credit.

DISCLOSURE OF CONFLICTS OF INTEREST

The EOCME assesses conflict of interest with its instructors, faculty, planners, and other individuals who are in a position to control the content of CME activities. All relevant conflicts of interest that are identified are thoroughly vetted by EOCME for fair balance, scientific objectivity, and patient care recommendations. EOCME is committed to providing its learners with CME activities that promote improvements or quality in healthcare and not a specific proprietary business or a commercial interest.

The planning committee, staff, authors and editors listed below have identified no financial relationships or relationships to products or devices they or their spouse/life partner have with commercial interest related to the content of this CME activity:

Denise Aloisio, MD; Kandy Bahadur, MD, FAAP; Meera S. Beharry, MD, FSAHM; Kimberly Boller, PhD; Arturo Brito, MD, MPH; Randal Christensen, MD, MPH, FAAP; Thomas Demaria, PhD; Breanna Gentile, PhD; Rachel Gilgoff, MD, CCTP, FAAP; Samuel Gnanakumar; Perry N. Halkitis, PhD, MS, MPH; Marjorie Hogan, MD, FAAP; Kerry Holland; Aldina M. Hovde, MSW; Randye Huron, MD; Tiffani J. Johnson, MD, MSc; Steven Kairys, MD, MPH; Marilu Kelly, MSN, RN, CNE, CHCP; Kadiatou Koita, MD, MH-GHS; Kristen D. Krause, MPH; Lauren V. Kullmann; Nicole M. Leopardi, MD, FAAP; Anthony J. Maiolatesi, BA; Randi Mandelbaum, JD, LLM; Sara Silverio Marques, DrPH, MPH; Rajkumar Mayakrishnan, BSc, MBA; Shilpa Pai, MD, FAAP; David J. Schonfeld, MD, FAAP; Leena Singh, DrPH, MPH; Andrew Spaedy, MD; Victor Strasburger, MD, FAAP

The planning committee, staff, authors and editors listed below have identified financial relationships or relationships to products or devices they or their spouse/life partner have with commercial interest related to the content of this CME activity:

Stacy Doumas, MD: research support from Allergan, Otsuka America Pharmaceutical, Inc., Shire, and Teva Pharmaceutical Industries Ltd.

Ramon Solhkhah, MD, MBA: research support from Alkermes, Pfizer Inc, Synerx Pharma, LLC, and Shire; consultant/advisor and research support from Alexza and Galen Limited.

UNAPPROVED / OFF-LABEL USE DISCLOSURE

The EOCME requires CME faculty to disclose to the participants:

1. When products or procedures being discussed are off-label, unlabelled, experimental, and/or investigational (not US Food and Drug Administration [FDA] approved); and
2. Any limitations on the information presented, such as data that are preliminary or that represent ongoing research, interim analyses, and/or unsupported opinions. Faculty may discuss information about pharmaceutical agents that is outside of FDA-approved labelling. This information is intended solely for CME and is not intended to promote off-label use of these medications. If you have any questions, contact the medical affairs department of the manufacturer for the most recent prescribing information.

TO ENROLL

To enroll in the *Pediatric Clinics of North America* Continuing Medical Education program, call customer service at 1-800-654-2452 or sign up online at http://www.theclinics.com/home/cme. The CME program is available to subscribers for an additional annual fee of USD 300.00.

METHOD OF PARTICIPATION

In order to claim credit, participants must complete the following:

1. Complete enrolment as indicated above.
2. Read the activity.
3. Complete the CME Test and Evaluation. Participants must achieve a score of 70% on the test. All CME Tests and Evaluations must be completed online.

In order to claim MOC points, participants must complete the following:

1. Complete steps listed above for claiming CME credit
2. Provide your specialty board ID#, birth date (MM/DD), and attestation.
3. Online MOC submission is only available for the American Board of pediatrics' (ABP) Maintenance of Certification (MOC) program

CME INQUIRIES/SPECIAL NEEDS

For all CME inquiries or special needs, please contact elsevierCME@elsevier.com.

Contributors

CONSULTING EDITOR

BONITA F. STANTON, MD
Founding Dean, Hackensack Meridian School of Medicine at Seton Hall University, President, Academic Enterprise, Hackensack Meridian Health Robert C. and Laura C. Garrett Endowed Chair for the School of Medicine, Professor of Pediatrics, Nutley, New Jersey

EDITORS

ARTURO BRITO, MD, MPH
Executive Director, The Nicholson Foundation, Newark, New Jersey

STEVEN KAIRYS, MD, MPH
Chairman and Professor, Department of Pediatrics, Hackensack Meridian School of Medicine at Seton Hall, Nutley, New Jersey, USA; Department of Pediatrics, Jersey Shore University Medical Center, Neptune, New Jersey

AUTHORS

DENISE ALOISIO, MD
Chief, Division of Developmental Behavioral Pediatrics, Hackensack Meridian Health, K. Hovnanian Children's Hospital - Jersey Shore University Medical Center, Neptune, New Jersey; Assistant Professor of Pediatrics, Hackensack Meridian School of Medicine, Nutley, New Jersey

KANDY BAHADUR, MD, FAAP
General Pediatrician, Bridgewater, New Jersey

MEERA S. BEHARRY, MD, FSAHM
Adolescent Medicine, Section Chief, McLane Children's Medical Center, McLane Children's Specialty Clinic, Baylor Scott and White, Assistant Professor of Pediatrics, Texas A&M Health Science Center (Affiliate), Temple, Texas

KIMBERLY BOLLER, PhD
Chief Strategy and Evaluation Officer, The Nicholson Foundation, Newark, New Jersey

ARTURO BRITO, MD, MPH
Executive Director, The Nicholson Foundation, Newark, New Jersey

RANDAL CHRISTENSEN, MD, MPH, FAAP
President/Founder, Randal Christensen Consulting, LLC, Henderson, Nevada

THOMAS DEMARIA, PhD
National Center for School Crisis and Bereavement, Los Angeles, California

STACY DOUMAS, MD
Associate Professor and Vice Chair, Department of Psychiatry and Behavioral Health, Hackensack Meridian School of Medicine at Seton Hall University, Nutley, New Jersey; Vice Chair of Education, Department of Psychiatry, Jersey Shore University Medical Center, Neptune, New Jersey

BREANNA GENTILE, PhD
Researcher, Clinic + Research, Center for Youth Wellness, San Francisco, California

RACHEL GILGOFF, MD, CCTP, FAAP
Chief Medical Officer, Stronger Brains Inc, Former Director of Clinical Innovation and Research, Center for Youth Wellness, San Francisco, California

PERRY N. HALKITIS, PhD, MS, MPH
Center for Health, Identity, Behavior and Prevention Studies, Rutgers School of Public Health, Newark, New Jersey; Departments of Biostatistics and Urban-Global Health, Rutgers School of Public Health, Piscataway, New Jersey

MARJORIE HOGAN, MD, FAAP
Professor, Department of Pediatrics, University of Minnesota, Hennepin County Medical Center, Minneapolis, Minnesota

ALDINA M. HOVDE, MSW
Director, Safety and Trauma Informed Care Initiatives, New Jersey Chapter, American Academy of Pediatrics, East Windsor, New Jersey

RANDYE F. HURON, MD
Chief, Developmental and Behavioral Pediatrics, Director, Institute for Child Development, Hackensack Meridian Health, Joseph M. Sanzari, Children's Hospital - Hackensack University Medical Center, Hackensack, New Jersey; Assistant Professor of Pediatrics, Hackensack Meridian School of Medicine at Seton Hall University, Nutley, New Jersey

TIFFANI J. JOHNSON, MD, MSc
Assistant Professor of Emergency Medicine, University of California, Davis, Davis

STEVEN KAIRYS, MD, MPH
Chairman and Professor, Department of Pediatrics, Hackensack Meridian School of Medicine at Seton Hall, Nutley, New Jersey, USA; Department of Pediatrics, Jersey Shore University Medical Center, Neptune, New Jersey

KADIATOU KOITA, MD, MH-GHS, MS-GHS
Senior Clinical Research Manager, Clinic + Research, Center for Youth Wellness, San Francisco, California

KRISTEN D. KRAUSE, MPH
Center for Health, Identity, Behavior and Prevention Studies, Rutgers School of Public Health, Newark, New Jersey; Department of Health Behavior, Society, and Policy, Rutgers School of Public Health, Piscataway, New Jersey

LAUREN V. KULLMANN, BS
Medical Student, Rowan University, School of Osteopathic Medicine, Stratford, New Jersey

NICOLE M. LEOPARDI, MD, FAAP
General Pediatrician, Cooper University Healthcare, Children's Regional Center, Assistant Professor of Pediatrics, Assistant Director, Pediatrics Clerkship, CMSRU, Medical Director, Medical Home for Trafficked Minors, Children's Regional Center, Camden, New Jersey

ANTHONY J. MAIOLATESI, BA
Center for Health, Identity, Behavior and Prevention Studies, Rutgers School of Public Health, Newark, New Jersey; Department of Social and Behavioral Sciences, Yale School of Public Health, New Haven, Connecticut; Center for Interdisciplinary Research on AIDS, Yale University, New Haven, Connecticut

RANDI MANDELBAUM, JD, LLM
Distinguished Clinical Professor of Law, Annamay Sheppard Scholar, Director, Child Advocacy Clinic, Rutgers Law School, Newark, New Jersey

SARA SILVERIO MARQUES, DrPH, MPH
Director of Strategic Initiatives, Center for Youth Wellness, San Francisco, California

SHILPA PAI, MD, FAAP
Associate Professor of Pediatrics, Rutgers Robert Wood Johnson Medical School, New Brunswick, New Jersey

DAVID J. SCHONFELD, MD, FAAP
Director, National Center for School Crisis and Bereavement, Children's Hospital Los Angeles, Professor of Clinical Pediatrics, Keck School of Medicine of USC, Los Angeles, California

LEENA SINGH, DrPH, MPH
Program Director, National Pediatric Practice Community, Center for Youth Wellness, San Francisco, California

RAMON SOLHKHAH, MD, FHELA
Founding Chair and Professor, Department of Psychiatry and Behavioral Health, Hackensack Meridian School of Medicine at Seton Hall University, Nutley, New Jersey; Chair, Department of Psychiatry, Jersey Shore University Medical Center, Neptune, New Jersey

ANDREW SPAEDY, MD
Resident, Department of Psychiatry, Jersey Shore University Medical Center, Neptune, New Jersey

VICTOR STRASBURGER, MD, FAAP
Distinguished Professor of Pediatrics Emeritus, University of New Mexico School of Medicine, Albuquerque, New Mexico

Contents

Foreword: The Vulnerable Child   xv

Bonita F. Stanton

Preface: Addressing Challenges Facing Today's Children   xvii

Arturo Brito and Steven Kairys

Changing the Pediatric Paradigm: Focusing on Strengths   247

Arturo Brito and Kimberly Boller

> Pediatricians need to adopt a strengths-based approach within their practices to better address their patients' health-related social needs. This approach becomes even more important as the pediatric population in the United States becomes increasingly diverse. Pediatricians must be cognizant of and address biases within their practices to maximize effectiveness of a strengths-based approach. With evidence mounting about their significance to health, a paradigm shift is needed to address health-related social needs by focusing on assets, not deficits. This shift will hopefully improve pediatric health outcomes which have languished in the United States, despite outspending other wealthy nations for decades.

Adverse Childhood Experiences, Outcomes, and Interventions   259

Rachel Gilgoff, Leena Singh, Kadiatou Koita, Breanna Gentile, and Sara Silverio Marques

> Adverse childhood experiences (ACEs) are stressful or traumatic events that children experience before age 18 years. Studies have linked exposure to ACEs and negative health, and developmental and behavioral outcomes. Screening in pediatric medical settings provides a clear opportunity for early detection, intervention, and treatment. Providing anticipatory guidance on healthy relationships, sleep, exercise, nutrition, mindfulness, and nature is essential. Pediatric medical providers must screen and intervene. Primary care is the ideal setting for ACE screening because interacting with children and their families at regular intervals can allow patients and providers to develop a trusting relationship.

Twenty Questions (and Answers) About Media Violence and Cyberbullying   275

Marjorie Hogan and Victor Strasburger

> For decades, pediatricians have been concerned about the impact of media on the health and well-being of children and adolescents. Robust research has found an association between exposure to media violence and real-life aggression in children and teens. Other effects include desensitization, fear, and attitudes that violence is a means of resolving conflict. Ongoing research finds similar associations between exposure to video game violence and real-life attitude and behavior. Cyberbullying is an

emerging threat to youth. Parents, pediatricians, schools, and government all have roles to play to mitigate the potential harmful effects of violent media on children and teens.

The Health Challenges of Emerging Adult Gay Men: Effecting Change in Health Care   **293**

Perry N. Halkitis, Anthony J. Maiolatesi, and Kristen D. Krause

This article focuses on the health and health care challenges experienced by young and emerging adult gay men. Evidence is provided on the extent to which young and emerging adult gay men are disproportionally burdened by multidimensional health disparities, barriers to health care access, and inadequate provider-patient interactions. Recommendations are provided for health care providers and public health officials working with populations of emerging adult gay men that might have the greatest overall impact on improving this population's well-being and access to competent health care by increasing providers' awareness of the unique needs of young and emerging adult gay men.

Supporting Immigrant Children and Youth: What Pediatricians and Other Clinicians Can Do   **309**

Randi Mandelbaum

For migrant children, many obstacles stand in the way of them securing even the most basic of necessities, and many live with the constant threat of being returned to countries where their very lives are in danger. These children and families, many of whom have experienced multiple forms of trauma, both in their home countries and on the journey to the United States, have extensive needs (for medical, mental health, educational, and legal services) that are not being met. Although pediatric medical professionals cannot respond to all issues, they are well situated to assist these vulnerable children.

Child Abuse and Neglect: The Role of the Primary Care Pediatrician   **325**

Steven Kairys

Child abuse affects more than 10% of children in the United States. For most children it is the result of family dysfunction. Child abuse affects children from all socioeconomic classes. Pediatricians have an important role to play in prevention and early detection of abuse. There are sentinel injuries, now summarized as Clinical Prediction Rules that can guide the general pediatrician to take more definitive steps to suspect and report child abuse and neglect. Primary prevention should be part of the anticipatory guidance and support that pediatricians provide to all of their families.

Autism as Representative of Disability   **341**

Denise Aloisio and Randye F. Huron

Pediatricians care for many children with autism spectrum disorder who demonstrate a wide range of abilities and needs. This population is vulnerable because of lags in diagnosis, difficulty accessing services, overlooked medical conditions, behavioral difficulties during medical visits, parental stress, bullying, comorbid mental health issues, and variable transitional care moving from adolescence to young adulthood. Comprehensive care includes earlier recognition of symptoms with timely referral to early intervention services. It includes primary pediatricians partnering with the family, developmental pediatricians, and other specialists to reduce the vulnerabilities by medical advocacy, family education, and appropriate behavior intervention to improve functioning.

Homelessness in Pediatric Populations: Strategies for Prevention, Assistance, and Advocacy   357

Meera S. Beharry and Randal Christensen

Recent data indicate that homelessness among pediatric and adolescent populations is significantly higher than previous studies and point-in-time counts indicate. Pediatricians and other health care providers often see children and youth who are at risk of or are currently experiencing homelessness, but may not be aware of their status. This article summarizes current definitions of homelessness and data on common health issues for pediatric patients. Information on how to recognize and help those experiencing homelessness as well as areas for continued advocacy is shared.

Substance Use Disorders in Vulnerable Children   373

Andrew Spaedy, Stacy Doumas, and Ramon Solhkhah

Substance use remains a major challenge in adolescent health. The coexisting use of these substances often creates hurdles for accurate diagnosis of other comorbid psychiatric conditions. It is of critical importance that health care providers be aware of both the isolated presentation of substance use disorder and that with coexisting psychiatric illness in vulnerable children.

The Impact of Food Insecurity on Child Health   387

Shilpa Pai and Kandy Bahadur

Food insecurity (FI) has severe implications on children's health and their future health outcomes. Children with FI have limited access to healthy foods and demonstrate poorer eating behavior, leading to chronic absenteeism, school failure, and chronic disease. Given the health implications of FI, it is imperative for pediatricians to screen all children, and advocate for protecting necessary nutritional programs that exist to mitigate FI and for improved accessibility of nutritious, healthy food options, especially in locations labeled as food deserts. Given the severe consequences of FI, collaboration of multidisciplinary teams is necessary to facilitate enhanced care of all patients.

Supporting Children After School Shootings   397

David J. Schonfeld and Thomas Demaria

Anticipatory guidance should be provided to families on identifying and addressing common adjustment reactions after a school shooting. Although adjustment difficulties may be related to post-traumatic and grief reactions, many will not be directly attributable to the school shooting.

Understanding how to cope with associated worries and reactions can help children better adjust. Pediatricians can assist with guidance about the development of a reasonable timeline for emotional and academic recovery, traumatic stress/loss, coping strategies, support for students with special needs, identification of students most in need of support, identification of staff who are most likely impacted, and appropriate preparedness activities.

The Intersection of Child Trafficking and Health Care: Our Unique Role as Pediatric Clinicians   413

Nicole M. Leopardi, Aldina M. Hovde, and Lauren V. Kullmann

Human trafficking is a pervasive public health problem that affects children of all ages. Health care clinicians can play a unique role in identifying and intervening for trafficking victims through acknowledging biases, understanding the risk factors and red flags, and implementing a trauma-informed care approach in their clinics and institutions. It is through collaboration, education, and research that health care clinicians can work to recognize and respond to this crime perpetrated against the youngest and most vulnerable patients.

Racial Bias and Its Impact on Children and Adolescents   425

Tiffani J. Johnson

Racial bias is pervasive throughout society and can impact children and adolescents in the health care, education, and criminal justice systems. This article provides a state-of-the-science review of implicit bias in health care. It also reviews the evidence of how bias impacts children in other aspects of society, explores bias as it relates to the broader context of structural racism in America, and summarizes the impact of bias and discrimination on youth academic, behavioral, and health outcomes. Evidence-based strategies are provided to help pediatricians identify and confront their own personal biases.

PEDIATRIC CLINICS OF NORTH AMERICA

FORTHCOMING ISSUES

June 2020
Pediatric Prevention
Henry Roane, *Editor*

August 2020
Telehealth for Pediatricians
C. Jason Wang, Josip Car,
Barry S. Zuckerman, *Editors*

October 2020
Pediatric Cardiology
Dunbar D. Ivy, Pei-Ni Jone,
and Stephen R. Daniels, *Editors*

RECENT ISSUES

February 2020
Pediatric Orthopedics
Paul T. Haynes, *Editor*

December 2019
Substance Abuse
David R. Rosenberg and
Leslie H. Lundahl, *Editors*

October 2019
Pediatric Immunology and Allergy
Elizabeth Secord, *Editor*

SERIES OF RELATED INTEREST

Clinics in Perinatology
http://www.perinatology.theclinics.com/
Advances in Pediatrics
http://www.advancesinpediatrics.com/

THE CLINICS ARE AVAILABLE ONLINE!
Access your subscription at:
www.theclinics.com

Foreword
The Vulnerable Child

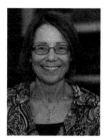

Bonita F. Stanton, MD
Consulting Editor

"The vulnerable child." A vague description, but one that commands the attention of any, and every, pediatrician, and virtually every child-care provider and parent. Pediatric education and practices are designed to identify potential vulnerabilities to mitigate, or eliminate, their impacts before any negative consequences for a child's development or life course can arise.

But, all of us who interact with children and families and child-care professionals understand the complexities, the variability, and the magnitude of efforts needed by a range of family, care providers, and health professionals needed to maximize the outcomes for each, and every, vulnerable child.

Further complicating this task are the total number and breadth of the range of the factors associated with child vulnerability. Furthermore, as we contemplate child vulnerability, we must remember that rarely is a child burdened by only 1 vulnerability and that the impact on a child of each additional vulnerability is more likely to be multiplicative rather than merely additive. As well, the nature, presentation, and significance of each vulnerability will change as a child ages or matures or struggles, and as the environment in which he or she is living changes.

In this issue of *Pediatric Clinics of North America*, the guest editors, Arturo Brito, MD and Steven Kairys, MD, have addressed this complex and important issue in a very thoughtful and constructive way. Rather than attempting to address all sources and expressions of vulnerability, they have elected to identify clusters of causes or manifestations of vulnerabilities, including those resulting from biologic (for example, "Autism as Representative of Disability"), social (for example, "Substance Use Disorders in Vulnerable Children"), economic (for example, "The Impact of Food Insecurity on Child Health"), or other environmental issues (for example, "Supporting Children After School Shootings," "Racial Bias and Its Impact on Children and Adolescents," "Supporting Immigrant Children and Youth: What Pediatricians and Other Clinicians Can Do," "The Intersection of Child Trafficking and Health Care: Our Unique Role as

https://doi.org/10.1016/j.pcl.2020.01.003
0031-3955/20/© 2020 Published by Elsevier Inc.

Pediatric Clinicians," and "Homelessness in Pediatric Populations: Strategies for Prevention, Assistance, and Advocacy"). The editors and authors describe a range of approaches to addressing these issues, reviewing evidence-based approaches backed by years of experience as well as several new approaches (see, for example, "Changing the Pediatric Paradigm: Focusing on Strengths").

The issues being addressed in this issue of *Pediatric Clinics of North America* are of great importance to all of us who care about children. Drs Brito, Kairys, and I anticipate, and hope, that you will find this information helpful in your roles as child-care providers.

Bonita F. Stanton, MD
Hackensack Meridian School of Medicine at Seton Hall University
Academic Enterprise
340 Kingsland Street, Building 123
Nutley, NJ 07110, USA

E-mail address:
bonita.stanton@shu.edu

Preface
Addressing Challenges Facing Today's Children

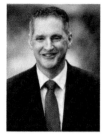 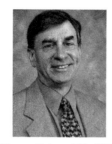

Arturo Brito, MD, MPH   Steven Kairys, MD, MPH
Editors

This issue of *Pediatric Clinics of North America* focuses on the many ways United States (US) children have become more vulnerable in the twenty-first century. The days of feeling safe in the streets and in school and having a parent at home after school with worries limited to experimenting with alcohol or cigarettes are long past. There have certainly always been problems, but the extent and high dose in today's world are extraordinary. A key to understanding the complexities of this rapidly changing environment is described in an article that demonstrates the connections between daily exposure to social and mass media and violence. And the age-old problem of substance use disorders is discussed in another article with a contemporary twist—a focus on vaping and the interplay of substance use with comorbid mental health disorders. Exacerbated by the pace of society and overreliance on technology, many of the specific concerns highlighted in this issue are done in the hopes of expanding the sensitivity and responsiveness of the pediatric community and to give some direction on how best to engage.

Investments in infrastructure within and peripheral to the health care system are mostly lacking for topics covered. Some, like human trafficking and homelessness, are generally not thought to be child related and therefore are often out of the purview of the field of pediatrics. In others, pediatricians often lack training to meet the needs of specific subpopulations, such as those of emerging young adult gay men or immigrant children. In the case of school shootings, one must be cognizant of their wide-ranging impact on the lifelong mental health of affected children, families, schools, and communities. In all of these scenarios, pediatricians have an opportunity, if not the responsibility, to have a sensitive and nuanced approach to reach and find the resilience that each child possesses.

Pediatricians are thereby positioned to lead the way so that *all* children are given the resources necessary to thrive. The opportunity to set foundational elements for lifelong

Pediatr Clin N Am 67 (2020) xvii–xviii
https://doi.org/10.1016/j.pcl.2020.01.002
0031-3955/20/© 2020 Published by Elsevier Inc.

pediatric.theclinics.com

health exists primarily for 2 reasons: (1) pediatricians by and large focus on prevention and healthy development and (2) pediatricians are generally trusted by parents and communities. However, to move the needle and help realize a health care system that serves not only children better but also all of society requires addressing the roots of much ill health in the US. Two articles in this issue are particularly focused on such onsets, one on adverse childhood experiences (ACEs), the other taking a deep dive at racism as well as implicit bias and institutional bias and their impact on child health. Despite research supporting the health care system tackling these topics, engagement on these issues remain elusive to most pediatric practices.

The field has even fallen short in resolving age-old problems that are relatively commonplace, though admittedly messy to incorporate into conventional practice. Examples detailed in this issue include child abuse (a subset of ACEs), food insecurity, and the challenges of meeting the needs of children with autism spectrum disorder. Authors for each of these articles share an emphasis on the importance of early detection and management to minimize lifelong impact to physical and mental health. Authors also acknowledge that family and social constructs make each condition more challenging for the pediatric practice and offer up practical solutions for linking these and other external factors to address more effectively. This same comprehensive approach should be applied to just about any complex challenge or condition in pediatrics.

The introductory article offers a broad framework for building on the innate and unique strengths of children, families, and communities, regardless of the issue being addressed. In approaching practice through this perspective, pediatricians will find themselves more satisfied with their work because of tangibly improved patient outcomes, which can lead the way for others toward a more effective health care system for all.

Arturo Brito, MD, MPH
The Nicholson Foundation
60 Park Place, 19th Floor
Newark, NJ 07102, USA

Steven Kairys, MD, MPH
Department of Pediatrics
Hackensack Meridian School of Medicine at Seton Hall
340 Kingsland Street
Nutley, NJ 07110, USA

E-mail addresses:
abrito@thenicholsonfoundation.org (A. Brito)
steven.kairys@hackensackmeridian.org (S. Kairys)

Changing the Pediatric Paradigm: Focusing on Strengths

Arturo Brito, MD, MPH*, Kimberly Boller, PhD

KEYWORDS

- Health-related social needs • Strengths-based approach • Physician bias
- Health disparities

KEY POINTS

- Pediatricians have been at the forefront in understanding how the social environment impacts health.
- Despite significantly higher spending compared with similar nations, the United States fares far worse in pediatric health outcomes.
- Ideologies meant to protect vulnerable populations, including children, have inadvertently led to stigmatization and, in some cases, worse outcomes.
- Adopting a strengths-based approach in pediatric practice increases the chances of improved outcomes for all patients.
- Pediatricians must also address their own biases to maximize effectiveness of a strengths-based approach.

INTRODUCTION

Pediatricians have long understood that children are by nature resilient. Some social and environmental conditions can, however, challenge resilience and compromise child health and well-being. A paradigm shift is needed in pediatric practice that builds on the strengths of children, families, and communities; the current health care system is simply not working to improve pediatric health. The United States spends more per capita on pediatric health care than any other country by far, yet mortality and morbidity rates have exceeded those of comparable nations for decades. One reason for this is that the incorporation of effective social programs into medical practice has been limited. As evidence mounts for the extent to which the social environment drives health outcomes, pediatricians should reevaluate their practices and incorporate available programs known to counter the negative impacts of poverty, food insecurity, lack of transportation, and other health-related social needs. To maximize

The Nicholson Foundation, 60 Park Place, 19th Floor, Newark, NJ 07102, USA
* Corresponding author.
E-mail address: abrito@thenicholsonfoundation.org
Twitter: @DrArturoNJ (A.B.); @KimBoller1 (K.B.)

Pediatr Clin N Am 67 (2020) 247–258
https://doi.org/10.1016/j.pcl.2019.12.010
0031-3955/20/© 2020 Elsevier Inc. All rights reserved.

effectiveness, pediatricians must adopt a strengths-based approach and engage in reflective practice to address potentially harmful biases. Together, this allows for greater focus on external factors rendering some children more vulnerable than others while building on assets, not deficits. The result will be improved health outcomes for patients and their communities, and a more fulfilling practice for the pediatrician.

BACKGROUND AND HISTORY
Beyond Clinical Walls

At its essence, pediatrics focuses on prevention, targets healthy development, and works within the context of family and community. Leaders in the field have long understood this. Dr Abraham Jacobi (1830–1919), considered to be the father of American pediatrics, encouraged physicians to advocate on behalf of children and foresaw the need for pediatricians to "sit in and control school boards, health departments, and legislatures."[1] Dr Jacobi recommended that pediatricians think about "all aspects of health," not just that which was disease based.[2]

The American Academy of Pediatrics (AAP) has endorsed the medical home model for decades, with the first known documentation of the term in the book, *Standards of Child Care*, published in 1967 by the AAP Council on Pediatric Practice. Although the term was originally used to describe a place to centralize medical records for children with special health care needs, the definition evolved over time and now refers to an approach.[3] As per the AAP,

> *A medical home is **not** a building or place; it extends beyond the walls of a clinical practice.[4]*

This approach requires developing partnerships with families to provide primary health care that is accessible, family centered, coordinated, comprehensive, continuous, compassionate, and culturally effective.[3]

Less than Desirable Outcomes

Evidence indeed supports the need for seeing beyond clinical walls. Despite spending more per capita on health care for children than any other country, the United States (US) has had the highest infant (up to the first birthday) and child (1–19 years of age) mortality rates since the 1980s and 1970s, respectively, among nations with similar levels of economic development and political structure.[5] Childhood morbidity rates in injury, obesity, HIV infection, and adolescent pregnancy are also worse in the US.[5]

The Institute of Medicine (IOM) report, *U.S. Health in International Perspective: Shorter Lives, Poorer Health*, emphasizes that although no single factor fully explains this health disadvantage, likely contributors include the following:

- A fragmented US health system with a large uninsured population;
- Risk behaviors that, compared with people of similar nations, include Americans' higher consumption of calories, less frequent use of seatbelts, more driving under the influence of alcohol and causing traffic accidents, higher gun ownership, and greater adolescent sexual activity with higher rates of unprotected sex; and
- Higher rates of poverty and income inequality with decreased access to safety net programs in the US compared with other wealthy nations.[6]

Each of these contributing factors is also influenced by physical and social environments unique to each community, such as limited access to healthy foods, decreased availability of contraception, lack of safe walking and play areas, or unaffordable and unhealthy housing.[6]

Health-Related Social Needs

Social, economic, and behavioral factors described in the IOM report help to explain why high levels of spending on health care are not aligned with better outcomes. By most estimates, medical care accounts for only 10% to 20% of the modifiable contributors to healthy outcomes for a population.[7] The other 80% to 90% come from social determinants of health (SDOH), health-related behaviors, and socioeconomic and environmental factors.[7] As defined by the World Health Organization, SDOH

> are the conditions in which people are born, grow, live, work and age. These are shaped by the distribution of money, power, and resources at global, national and local levels.[8]

SDOH are estimated to contribute from 40% to 60% of health outcomes,[9] affecting low-income populations more often because of their interrelatedness[10] to the economy, environment, and behavior. In fact, 60% of preventable deaths are rooted in modifiable behaviors and exposures that occur in the community.[11]

The federal Centers for Medicare and Medicaid Services (CMS) is currently evaluating the effectiveness of a 10-item screening tool of health-related social needs (HRSN), a core subset of SDOH, on health care costs and health outcomes. The tool, "designed to be short, accessible, consistent, and inclusive,"[12] originally included 5 core HRSN domains—housing instability, food insecurity, transportation needs, utility needs, and interpersonal safety.[13] The CMS selected these domains because of existing evidence linking each to poor health or increased health care use and cost, ability of community service providers to meet the identified need, and health care providers not addressing the need systemically.[12] In the final version of the screening tool, questions from 8 other domains were added—financial strain, employment, family and community support, education, physical activity, substance use, mental health, and disabilities.[14]

The additions of financial strain, employment, and education are consistent with a study by Garg and colleagues[15] of mothers of healthy infants attending urban community health centers. Among 6 basic needs assessed, participants in this study self-identified the following, in order of frequency: unemployment (57%), housing (43%), child care (29%), food insecurity (20%), inadequate parental education (17%), and home heating (9%). Decades of research have in fact revealed that educational status, especially of the mother, is a major predictor of health outcomes[16] and, at least in the US, health benefits associated with increased educational attainment have sharply expanded over recent decades.[17,18] The study by Garg and colleagues[15] had significant and encouraging results—a 1-year follow-up comparing study participants with those receiving usual health care services demonstrated that study mothers were more likely to be enrolled in a new community resource and employed, study children were more likely to be enrolled in child care, and study families had greater odds of receiving fuel assistance and lower odds of being homeless.

PREVALENCE
Poverty

Children are the poorest group in the US.[19] In 2018, approximately 16% of children (<18 years of age) in the US were living below the federal poverty level (FPL). In 2018, the FPL was a $25,100 annual income for a family of 4 living in the 48 contiguous states,[20] representing 11.9 million children.[21] Historically, there has been wide variation in child poverty between states, from 10% in New Hampshire to 30% in Mississippi for 2018. In the same year, an estimated 39%

of children were living at less than 200% ($50,200[20]) of the federal poverty level, the marker generally used to identify low-income families. Again, there was wide variation, from 24% in New Hampshire to 52% in both Mississippi and New Mexico.[22]

However, the greatest variation in child poverty is seen by race and ethnicity. In 2018, disparities between non-Hispanic white children (11% poverty rate) and some minority groups was more than 25% points. For example, 32% of African American, 31% of Native American, and 26% of Latino children lived in poverty.[23]

Economic Instability as a Social Determinant

Increasingly, researchers are looking at stability as a contributor to children's well-being, and the absence of it—instability—as more than a risk factor for compromised child health and well-being outcomes. Instead of simply quantifying one aspect of stability, such as consistency in family income and reduction of economic shocks to the family, frameworks for documenting and quantifying stability provide insights to the multidetermined pathways to children's vulnerability. One definition of instability is "the experience of abrupt and/or involuntary change in individual, family, or community circumstances, which can have adverse implications for children's development."[24] Economic instability, also referred to as economic insecurity, is associated with other types of instability, including access to early care and education services that support parent employment, changes in household composition, and features such as whether parents are married or not, and a range of other characteristics that are commonly categorized as SDOH.[25]

Federal and state policy and program requirements may buffer or exacerbate the experience of instability in children's lives. For example, across states, families take up childcare subsidies through the Child Care Development Fund at different rates that are associated with factors, such as the burden on families of maintaining income eligibility for the program. In 7 states or territories, parents must go through a redetermination of eligibility every 6 months compared with 49 other states or territories that provide eligibility for 12 months at a time.[26] The churn families experience in entering and exiting programs because of changes in eligibility increases family stress and also decreases the continuity of child care that supports children's experiences of nurturing care by a small number of adults.[27]

A Diverse and Complex Population

Pediatricians today need to be prepared to meet the needs of a more diverse population and one with significant numbers of children and youth with mental and physical disabilities:

- Based on 2018 data, the majority of the country's children under 15 years of age are for the first time and the foreseeable future from groups that were formerly considered ethnic and racial minorities (Hispanic, black, Asian, and American Indian/Alaska Natives). In fact, children who are white are currently the minority in 14 states and the District of Columbia.[28]
- Between the 2011 to 2012 and 2017 to 2018 school years, the number of US public school students served under the 1975 Individuals with Disabilities Education Act—enacted to ensure free and appropriate public education and related services for children diagnosed with disabilities negatively impacting academic performance—increased from 6.4 million (13% of enrolled students) to 7.0 million (14%).[29]

- In 2016, among US children 3 to 17 years of age, 7.1% were diagnosed with anxiety disorders, 7.4% with a behavioral or conduct problem, and 3.2% with depression.[30]
- Approximately 16.8% of children and youths between 2 and 20 years of age are obese (body mass index at or greater than the 95th percentile for age and gender).[31]

Health Disparities

As defined by Kilbourne and colleagues,

Health disparities are observed clinically and statistically significant differences in health outcomes or health care use between socially distinct vulnerable and less vulnerable populations that are not explained by the effects of selection bias.[9]

In the US, people of color, sexual minorities, and those with disabilities tend to have reduced health care access and receive less quality of care[32] compared with their counterparts. Examples of health disparities include:

- Black and American Indian/Alaska Native women are more than 3 and 2 times likely, respectively, to die around pregnancy than white women.[33]
- Infant mortality rates for non-Hispanic blacks and American Indian/Alaska Natives are more than and nearly twice, respectively, that of non-Hispanic white children.[34]
- Children with special health care needs are more likely to be obese than other children.[35]
- Lesbian, gay, bisexual, and transgender people suffer more from mental health, substance abuse, and sexually transmitted diseases than the general population.[36]

Physician Bias

Although the factors that contribute to these and other health disparities are many, complex, and intermingled, research in recent decades is demonstrating that physician implicit bias—unconscious thoughts and feelings that are often automatically activated and influence behavior[32]—adds to the problem. This is the topic of Tiffani J. Johnson's article, "Racial Bias and Its Impact on Children and Adolescents," elsewhere in this issue. In her article, the author emphasizes that implicit attitudes favoring whites over blacks and Hispanics are similar for health care providers and the general population. And although her article focuses on racial bias, Johnson points out that other groups experience bias. This includes, for instance, members of the lesbian, gay, bisexual, and transgender community[36] and people who are obese.[37] That physician attitudes are no different than the general population is backed up by studies like that of Burke and colleagues,[36] where they found that 82% of heterosexual first-year medical students in a large US sample held at least some degree of implicit bias against gay and lesbian individuals. Regardless of the group, physician implicit bias has been found to contribute to health disparities[9] by affecting communication, treatment decisions, and adherence to provider recommendations.[32] What this means for pediatricians is that how they behave toward children and their parents may be influenced by negative stereotypes and biases that translate into care that is lower in quality and less warm and accepting for some families.

Stereotypes of specific groups as less than status in the minds of health care professionals have been inadvertently and ironically reinforced through an oversimplification and misinterpretation of the concept of vulnerability in the research field. Although the 3 principles—respect for persons, beneficence, and justice—of the 1978 *Belmont Report: Ethical Principles and Guidelines for the Protection of Human Subjects Research (Belmont Report)*[38] have "permeated" clinical care and have had largely positive and lasting impact in medical education and health care,[39] in their translation into research regulations certain populations were deemed categorically vulnerable.[40]

This oversimplification fails to account for the impact external factors and their complex and dynamic interactions with endogenous characteristics that, together, cause human behavior to change from conception to death. This malleability over time means that categorizing children and families in ways that can limit their potential for growth and learning is a disservice and only reinforces negative outcomes.[41] For example, pediatricians who make quick assumptions about the causes of a child's lack of sociability or cognitive skills and link child well-being to parent behavior without understanding parent experience and family circumstances may reduce a parent's feelings of efficacy and harm the parent–child relationship rather than help them to address any social or physical issues. Viewing parents in their developmental niche is as important as viewing their children.

SOLUTIONS

Pediatric practices should use a strengths-based approach to incorporate screening and referral protocols for HRSN.[11] This approach applies to all children, but is particularly important for those living in more challenging, discriminatory, or unstable environments. Understanding the holistic experiences of children and families and working to stabilize them through high-quality screening of strengths and needs and referral to community resources can mitigate the negative effects of chaotic and destabilizing experiences.

Engaging in Reflective Practice

However, as a part of the process of implementing a strengths-based approach, pediatricians and practice staff should engage in reflective practice to discover how interactions with children and families align with stated goals about how to support the parent–child bond, manage provider responses to family needs, and incorporate professional values, including equity. Reflective supervision, a practice used widely in the field of infant mental health, involves supervisors supporting clinicians in their work with children and families. By providing time for clinicians to problem solve together and address any secondary trauma, reflective supervision helps to avoid and address staff burnout.[42] Another form of reflective practice includes pediatricians and practice staff taking formalized and validated tests that will bring their biases to consciousness, such as the Implicit Association Test,[a] as described by Johnson in her article. The Implicit Association Test offers a series of tests in pediatric-relevant categories—gender, skin tone, sexuality, religion, disability, weight, age, and specific racial and ethnic groups. To the extent possible, others within the larger health care system supporting the practice should be encouraged to participate. It is important to emphasize that the intent is not to rid anyone of their biases, because that would be unrealistic for such ingrained thinking, but rather to bring these biases to the surface and minimize their impact. Reflective supervision can also be used to help staff use the results of such assessments, set goals toward overcoming them, and assess progress.

---

[a] https://implicit.harvard.edu/implicit/takeatest.html.

Integrating a Strengths-Based Approach

Integrating proven strengths-based models means working in partnership with children, families, and communities, drawing on their collective strengths to identify roadmaps for preventing, managing, and healing from disease. This is consistent with the medical home model as described by the AAP,

> A medical home builds partnerships with clinical specialists, families, and community resources. The medical home recognizes the family as a constant in a child's life and emphasizes partnership between health care professionals and families.[43]

In screening for child development, for example, the AAP emphasizes that a strengths-based approach offers a broader perspective, encourages health-promoting interactions, acknowledges that parents are experts on their family and want to do what is best for their child, complements shared decision making, and is more efficacious than the more often used deficit model, which focuses on problems.[44]

Boynton-Jarrett and Flacks use the *Strengthening Families* framework and its 5 protective factors—parental resilience, social connections, knowledge of parenting and child development, concrete support in times of need, and social and emotional competence of children[45]—to make 6 recommendations for operationalizing a strengths-based approach: (1) involving families and communities in the development of screening tools and protocols; (2) screening for both risk and protective factors; (3) setting realistic, family-driven screening priorities for HRSN; (4) ensuring screening is administered by team members trained and supervised in strengths-based approaches; (5) recognizing that social needs screening is not risk free for families; and (6) acknowledging family-level risks and strengths in a broader historical context.[13]

Addressing Health-Related Social Needs

Through a strengths-based approach, pediatricians should build partnerships with leadership from proven social programs, educational systems, public health agencies, and other community-based organizations that can address HRSN. The HRSN originally selected by CMS and those evaluated by Garg and colleagues—namely, housing instability, food insecurity, transportation needs, utility needs, interpersonal safety, child care access, parent education, and employment—are a good starting point. Others may be added as the formal process identifies unique needs of the practice population.

Boynton-Jarrett and Flacks highlight the importance of avoiding unintended consequences, such as undermining trust, by ensuring that screening for HRSN is person centered, integrated with referral and linkage to community-based resources, done within the context of a comprehensive systems approach, not limiting screening practices based on documented or assumed membership in particularly social groups, and acknowledging and building on family strengths.[46] HRSN are otherwise unlikely to be brought to the attention of pediatricians, primarily because most families do not recognize them as relevant to medical care or, when they do, are often fraught with shame. Therefore, screening for HRSN should become routine care for all practice patients and related information should be considered confidential and private, in line with how other medical information is customarily handled.

In choosing a tool for screening for HRSN through a strengths-based approach, pediatricians should consider the following: (1) capacity to address specific needs; (2) availability of local resources/referral networks; (3) ease of use within the practice; and (4) ability to capture specific needs.[47]

Incorporating into Technology

The chosen tool should be incorporated into the practice's electronic health record (EHR). Although financial challenges, lack of pediatric-specific functionalities, privacy concerns, and organizational and technical barriers persist in their use,[48] EHRs have become the norm in medical practice. In 1 study of US office-based pediatric practices, EHR use increased rose from 58% to 94% between 2009 and 2016. Just as important, during that span pediatricians became more likely to report improved EHR functionality (eg, increased availability of features like viewing laboratory results and ordering prescriptions electronically) and EHRs having a major positive impact on their practice.[48]

Incorporating HRSN screening-and-referral protocols into EHRs increases efficiency, normalizes them as part of the medical practice, provides opportunity for subsequent analysis of individual and the practice population, and has the potential to contribute to the financial viability of the practice through payor reimbursement. The tools best to incorporate meet the inclusion criteria described in the IOM report, *Capturing Social and Behavioral Domains and Measures in Electronic Health Records: Phase 2:*

- Strength of the evidence of the association of the domain with health;
- Usefulness of the domain, as measured for the individual, population, and research;
- Availability and standard representation of a reliable and valid measure(s) of the domain;
- Feasibility in terms of burdens placed on the patient and clinical care team, including time and costs;
- Sensitivity, such as the comfort of revealing personal information; and
- Accessibility of data from another source.[49]

Pediatricians should work with their EHR vendors, chief information officers, or other information technology staff to add selected HRSN in standardized format to their practices. Standardization facilitates clinical use, opportunity for tracking individual and practice encounters, and payor reimbursement, when available.

Considering Practice Staffing

Pediatricians and practice staff face many demands on their time, challenging optimal patient care. It is, therefore, unreasonable and arguably irresponsible to expect pediatricians to take on the role of screening and referring for HRSN. One practical and potentially fiscally advantageous solution is to employ a trained and certified community health worker (CHW)—a frontline public health worker trusted by and with insight into the community served.[50]

In some states, private and public payors are moving forward with reimbursement for certified CHWs to help practices and health care systems address HRSN. As of 2018, in an unpublished review of websites by The Nicholson Foundation, 17 states were providing Medicaid reimbursement for CHWs through varied mechanisms, some more expansive than others. Sixteen states also had voluntary CHW certification programs and boards.[b] It then behooves pediatricians to learn about their own states' Medicaid and major payors' current and forthcoming reimbursement policies.

---

[b] Acknowledgment: Review conducted by Wesley Wei, Public Health Policy Fellow, The Nicholson Foundation.

SUMMARY

Pediatricians have long understood that children are by nature resilient and that factors outside the clinical walls often impact overall health and well-being more than medical interventions. As research around HRSN builds, so too does interest in identifying protocols that can most effectively address them within clinical walls. In pediatrics, this means first identifying provider and institutional biases, which may themselves be detrimental to patient health and that are a prerequisite to incorporating protocols which screen for HRSN and link patients to relevant community services. The need to address systemic racism and bias in pediatric care is bolstered by changes in the demographics of children in the US. The approach to identifying and managing HRSN should be strength based and not focus on deficits or categorization of individuals into vaguely defined groups. To improve efficiency, pediatricians should work toward identifying their patients' biggest social challenges, build partnerships with proven and relevant community-based organizations, incorporate chosen protocols into the practice EHR system, and consider hiring CHWs best suited to work within the community and help families link to needed services.

ACKNOWLEDGMENTS

The authors would like to acknowledge the assistance of Kevin McManemin, MS, Communications Manager, The Nicholson Foundation, and Madison McHugh, MA, MBA, Communications Fellow, The Nicholson Foundation. Both provided substantial editing to this article.

DISCLOSURE

The authors have nothing to disclose.

REFERENCES

1. Ligon-Borden BL. Abraham Jacobi, MD: father of American pediatrics and advocate for children's health. Semin Pediatr Infect Dis 2003;14(3):245–9.
2. Available at: https://www.nursing.upenn.edu/nhhc/home-care/late-nineteenth-and-early-century-pediatrics/. Accessed October 16, 2019.
3. Sia C, Tonniges TF, Osterhus E, et al. History of the medical home concept. Pediatrics 2004;113:1473–8.
4. Available at: https://medicalhomeinfo.aap.org/overview/Pages/Whatisthemedicalhome.aspx. Accessed October 16, 2019.
5. Thakrar AP, Forrest AD, Maltenfort MG, et al. Child mortality in the US and 19 OECD comparator nations: a 50-year time-trend analysis. Health Aff 2018; 37(1):140–9.
6. National Research Council Institute of Medicine. U.S. health in international perspective: shorter lives, poorer health. Washington, DC: National Academies Press; 2013.
7. Magnan S. Social determinants of health 101 for health care: five plus five. NAM Perspectives. Washington, DC: National Academy of Medicine; 2017. p. 1–9. Discussion paper Available at: https://nam.edu/social-determinants-of-health-101-for-health-care-five-plus-five.
8. Available at: http://www.who.int/social_determinants/sdh_definition/en/. Accessed December 19, 2019.

9. Kilbourne AM, Switzer G, Hyman K, et al. Advancing health disparities research within the health care system: a conceptual framework. Am J Public Health 2006; 96(12):2113–21.

10. Berkowitz SA, Hulberg AC, Hong C, et al. Addressing basic resource needs to improve primary care quality: a community collaboration programme. BMJ Qual Saf 2016;25(3):164–72.

11. Alley DE, Asomugha CN, Conway PH, et al. Accountable Health Communities—addressing social needs through Medicare and Medicaid. N Engl J Med 2016; 374(1):8–11.

12. Billioux A, Verlander K, Anthony S, et al. Standardized screening for health-related social needs in clinical settings: the accountable health communities screening tool. Matinal Academy of Medicine, Washington, DC. Discussion paper. Available at: https://nam.edu/wp-content/uploads/2017/05/Standardized - Screening-for-Health-Related-Social-Needs-in-Clinical-Settings.pdf. Accessed November 22, 2019.

13. Boynton-Jarrett R, Flacks J. Strengths-based approaches to screening families for health-related social needs in the healthcare setting. Washington, DC: MLPB and the Center for the Study of Social Policy; 2018.

14. Accountable health communities health-related social needs screening tool, pdf downloaded from. Available at: https://innovation.cms.gov/initiatives/ahcm. Accessed December 13, 2019.

15. Garg A, Toy S, Trippodis Y, et al. Addressing social determinants of health at well child care visits: a cluster RCT. Pediatrics 2015;135(2):1–9.

16. Zimmerman E, Woolf SH. Understanding the relationship between education and health. Washington, DC: Institute of medicine; 2014. Discussion paper, Available at: http://www/iom.edu/understandingthereltionship. Accessed December 11, 2019.

17. Goldman D, Smith JP. The increasing value of education to health. Soc Sci Med 2011;72:1728–37.

18. IOM (Institute of Medicine). Exploring opportunities for collaboration between health and education to improve population health: workshop summary. Washington, DC: The National Academics Press; 2015. p. 1–2. Chapter 1.

19. De Navas-Walt C, Proctor BD, Smith JC, U.S. Census Bureau. Current population reports, P60-243, income, poverty, and health insurance coverage in the United States: 2012. Washington, DC: US Government Printing Office; 2013.

20. Available at: https://familiesusa.org/resources/federal-poverty-guidelines/. Accessed December 12, 2019.

21. Semega J, Kollar M, Creamer J, et al, U.S. Census Bureau. Current population reports, P60-266, income and poverty in the United States: 2018. Washington, DC: U.S. Government Printing Office; 2019.

22. Available at: https://datacenter.kidscount.org/data/tables/43-children-in-poverty# detailed/1/any/false/37,871,870,573,869,36,868,867,133,38/any/321,322. Accessed December 12, 2019.

23. The Annie E Casey Foundation. 2019 kids count data book: state trends in child well-being. Baltimore (MD): The Annie E. Casey Foundation; 2019. Available at: www.aecf.org/databook. Accessed November 19, 2019.

24. Adams G, Bogle M, Isaacs JB, et al. Stabilizing children's lives: insights for research and action. Washington, DC: Urban Institute; 2016.

25. Sandstrom H, Sandra H. The negative effects of instability on child development: a research synthesis. Washington, DC: Urban Institute; 2013. Available at: http://urbn.is/2d5OJNZ.

26. Tran V, Minton S, Haldar S, et al. Child care subsidies under the CCDF program: an overview of policy differences across states and territories as of October 1, 2016. OPRE report 2018-02. Washington, DC: Office of Planning, Research, and Evaluation, Administration for Children and Families, U.S. Department of Health and Human Services; 2018.

27. Sosinsky L, Ruprecht K, Horm D, et al. Including relationship based care practices in infant-toddler care: implications for practice and policy. brief prepared for the office of planning, research and evaluation, administration for children and families. Washington, DC: U.S. Department of Health and Human Services; 2016.

28. Frey WH. Less than half of children under 15 are white, census shows. Washington, DC: Brookings Institution; 2019. Available at: https://www.brookings.edu/research/less-than-half-of-us-children-under-15-are-white-census-shows/.

29. Available at: https://nces.ed.gov/programs/coe/indicator_cgg.asp. Accessed December 13, 2019.

30. Ghandour RM, Sherman LJ, Vladutiu CJ, et al. Prevalence and treatment of depression, anxiety, and conduct problems among US children. J Pediatr 2019;206:256–67.

31. Stanford FC, Kyle TK. Respectful language and care in childhood obesity. JAMA Pediatr 2018;172(11):1001–2.

32. Hall WJ, Chapman MV, Lee KM, et al. Implicit racial/ethnic bias among health care professionals and its influence on health care outcomes: a systematic review. Am J Public Health 2015;105(12):e60–76.

33. Petersen EE, Davis NL, Goodman D, et al. Racial/ethnic disparities in pregnancy-related deaths — United States, 2007–2016. MMWR Morb Mortal Wkly Rep 2019; 68:762–5.

34. Available at: https://www.cdc.gov/reproductivehealth/maternalinfanthealth/infantmortality.htm. Accessed December 16, 2019.

35. Available at: https://www.cdc.gov/ncbddd/disabilityandhealth/obesity.html. Accessed December 24, 2019.

36. Burke SE, Dovidio JF, Przedworski JM, et al. Do contact and empathy mitigate bias against gay and lesbian people among heterosexual first-year medical students? A report from the medical student CHANGE Study. Acad Med 2015;90(5): 549–52.

37. Chapman EN, Kaatz A, Carnes M. Physicians and implicit bias: how doctors may unwittingly perpetuate health care disparities. J Gen Intern Med 2013;28(11): 1504–10.

38. National Commission for the Protection of Human Subjects of Biomedical and Behavioral Research. The Belmont report: ethical principles and guidelines for the protection of human subjects of research. Bethesda (MD): US Government Printing Office; 1978.

39. Cassell EJ. The principles of the Belmont report revisited: how have respect for persons, beneficence, and justice been applied to clinical medicine? Hastings Cent Rep 2000;30(4):12–21.

40. Available at: https://www.hhs.gov/ohrp/regulations-and-policy/regulations/common-rule/index.html. Accessed November 28, 2019.

41. Halfon N, Larson K, Lu M, et al. Lifecourse health development: past, present and future. Matern Child Health J 2014;18:344–65.

42. Available at: https://www.zerotothree.org/resources/412-three-building-blocks-of-reflective-supervision. Accessed November 19, 2019.

43. Available at: https://medicalhomeinfo.aap.org/overview/Pages/Whatisthemedical-home.aspx. Accessed November 19, 2019.

44. Available at: https://www.aap.org/en-us/advocacy-and-policy/aap-health-initiatives/HALF-Implementation-Guide/communicating-with-families/pages/Strength-Based-Approach.aspx. Accessed December 24, 2019.

45. Available at: https://cssp.org/our-work/project/strengthening-families/. Accessed November 19, 2019.

46. Garg A, Boynton-Jarrett R, DWorkin PH. Avoiding the unintended consequences of a screening for social determinants of health. JAMA 2016;316(8):813.

47. Thomas-Henkel C, Schulman M. Screening for social determinants of health in populations with complex needs: implementation considerations. Center for Health Care Strategies, Inc. Brief; 2017.

48. Available at: https://www.aappublications.org/news/2019/03/07/research030719. Accessed November 28, 2019.

49. Institute of Medicine. Capturing social and behavioral domains and measures in electronic health records: phase 2. Washington, DC: The National Academies Press; 2014.

50. Available at: https://nachw.org/about/. Accessed December 13, 2019.

Adverse Childhood Experiences, Outcomes, and Interventions

Rachel Gilgoff, MD, CCTP[a], Leena Singh, DrPH, MPH[b],
Kadiatou Koita, MD, MH-GHS, MS-GHS[a], Breanna Gentile, PhD[a],*,
Sara Silverio Marques, DrPH, MPH[c]

KEYWORDS

- Adverse childhood experiences • Toxic stress • Pediatric stress • ACEs
- Pediatric trauma • Stress outcomes • Pediatric interventions

KEY POINTS

- Adverse childhood experiences (ACEs) are stressful or potentially traumatic events that children experience before age 18 years.
- In children and adolescents, numerous studies have linked exposure to ACEs and negative health, and developmental and behavioral outcomes.
- Screening in pediatric medical settings provides a clear opportunity for early detection, intervention, and treatment of children at risk for accumulating ACEs.
- Providing anticipatory guidance helps patients/caregivers understand ACEs and toxic stress and be attuned to the types of situations that may be causing stress for a child.
- Because ACEs are a risk factor for health conditions, it is incumbent on pediatric medical providers to screen and intervene.

INTRODUCTION

Adverse childhood experiences (ACEs) are stressful or potentially traumatic events that children experience before age 18 years. The term ACEs was coined in 1998 following the publication of the Adverse Childhood Experiences study (ACE study). ACEs are grouped into 3 domains: abuse, neglect, and household dysfunction, and include 10 categories of adverse experiences.[1,2]

[a] Clinic + Research, Center for Youth Wellness, 3450 Third Street, Building 2, Suite 201, San Francisco, CA 94124, USA; [b] National Pediatric Practice Community, Center for Youth Wellness, 3450 Third Street, Building 2, Suite 201, San Francisco, CA 94124, USA; [c] Center for Youth Wellness, 3450 Third Street, Building 2, Suite 201, San Francisco, CA 94124, USA
* Corresponding author.
E-mail address: bgentile@centerforyouthwellness.org

Pediatr Clin N Am 67 (2020) 259–273
https://doi.org/10.1016/j.pcl.2019.12.001
0031-3955/20/© 2019 Elsevier Inc. All rights reserved.

HISTORY AND BACKGROUND

Numerous studies have shown that ACEs, such as abuse, neglect, and household dysfunction, are common and associated in a dose-dependent manner with worse health outcomes.[1,3,4] Exposure to these ACEs without a positive adult relationship as buffer can lead to a toxic stress response in children, leading to higher risk for health and behavioral problems. The toxic stress response, characterized by a chronic dysregulation of the neuroendocrine and immune system via the hypothalamic-pituitary axis (HPA), leads to multisystemic alterations, resulting in changes to the body's metabolic and epigenetic functioning, and onset of diseases.[5] Exposure to adversity early in life, particularly during sensitive periods of child and adolescent development, is especially problematic because of enhanced sensitivity and likelihood of permanent and long-term integration into regulatory biological processes[6] (**Fig. 1**).

EPIDEMIOLOGY AND OTHER DATA

In adults, ACEs have been found to have a strong, dose-response association with cardiovascular disease, chronic lung disease, cancer, diabetes, headaches, autoimmune disease, sleep disturbances, early death, obesity, smoking, general poor health, depression, posttraumatic stress disorder (PTSD), anxiety, substance abuse, sexual risk taking, mental ill health, and interpersonal and self-directed violence.[7,8]

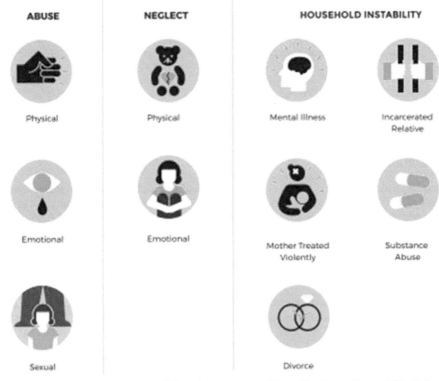

Fig. 1. The 3 types of adverse childhood experiences. (*From* The Truth About ACEs. Robert Woodson Foundation. Available at: https://www.rwjf.org/en/library/infographics/the-truth-about-aces.html. Copyright 2013. Robert Wood Johnson Foundation. Used with permission from the Robert Wood Johnson Foundation.)

In children and adolescents, numerous studies have linked exposure to ACEs and negative health, developmental and behavioral outcomes, including asthma, recurrent infections, cognitive and developmental delays, obesity, failure to thrive, and sleep disturbance,[9] as well as delinquent behavior, bullying, physical fighting, dating violence, and weapon carrying.[10–14] Researchers in the field continue to explore the relationship between other early childhood events and circumstances on children's health. Some of these adversities include hardship, serious illness, and death in the household.[15]

At the population level, the Behavioral Risk Factors Surveillance System (BRFSS), which has been collecting abuse and household dysfunction data in up to 42 states and District of Columbia, found that about two-thirds of the US population have been exposed to 1 or more ACEs. The data found ACEs to be associated with the following negative outcomes: traumatic injuries, depression, anxiety, suicide, PTSD, unintended pregnancy, pregnancy complications, fetal death, HIV, sexually transmitted diseases, cancer, diabetes, alcohol and drug abuse, unsafe sex, low educational level (noncompletion of high school), unemployment, and household poverty.[16] Like the ACE Study findings, the BRFSS data showed a graded dose-response relationship indicating that the risk of negative outcomes increased with the number of ACEs. This demonstrates that most people, irrelevant of socioeconomic, racial, and cultural background, are affected by some level of ACEs. This widespread exposure is why public health leaders and child advocates have called the unaddressed exposure to ACEs a public health crisis.

ROLE OF THE PEDIATRICIAN

The vast majority of children in the United States will see a pediatric provider 15 times for well child visits during the first 5 years of their life (Bright Futures/AAP Recommendations for Preventive Pediatric Health Care [Periodicity Schedule]). This time period is considered a valuable teaching opportunity for health care providers to support caregivers in promoting healthy practices for optimal child development. The case for the role of pediatric providers in addressing one of the most serious and consequential early life circumstances—that of exposure to childhood adversity has been established.[17,18] This dire public health issue is met with promise, but also precaution due to lack of provider training and time. Even so, pediatric providers are invested in exploring how they can improve the long-term trajectory of children's lives through screening and treatment. This written perspective highlights actionable next steps for pediatric providers in pursuit of science-informed clinical practices to address child adversity and toxic stress and focuses on ACEs as risk factors for toxic stress.

The perspective in this article is provided in 3 sections: (1) ACEs screening in pediatrics, (2) anticipatory guidance and domains of intervention, and (3) resources and referrals.

Adverse Childhood Experiences Screening in Pediatrics

Screening in pediatric medical settings provides a clear opportunity for early detection, intervention and treatment of children at risk for accumulating ACEs.[19] An ACEs screen is not designed to be an in-depth assessment of child abuse but, rather, to provide an assessment of a child's risk for developing neuroendocrine and immune dysregulation, referred to as a toxic stress response. This provides the health care provider and team with valuable information that can help inform clinical management of illness.

Although initial ACE research pointed to the associations between ACEs and adult health, more recent research demonstrated child behavioral and health outcomes associated with ACEs, making screening in pediatrics essential to curb further disease.[9,20] In addition, the substantial individual variability in how early adversity and toxic stress manifests over the life course, and the varied presentations of toxic stress physiology, make universally screening all pediatric patients for risk of toxic stress essential—even for those who may not be obviously symptomatic.[6]

Published studies show that caregivers are receptive to ACEs screening and feel comfortable discussing ACEs with their pediatricians as long as there is a trusting relationship.[15,21] Parents find the topic of ACEs to be of value to their child's care and are also largely unaware that ACEs can have lasting health impacts from exposure under the age of 5 years (*CYW Market Research, 2017. Unpublished data*).

Screening also provides an opportunity for clinicians to support parents and caregivers to be buffers for their children, especially those with high exposure to adversity. This is critical as the evidence suggests that one effective intervention in preventing the negative outcomes associated with ACEs is a caring supportive adult.[22,23] By exploring the protective and risk factors that are affecting the health of patients and families in the primary care setting, medical providers can help tap into existing sources of resilience, promote parent-child attachment, and enhance the protective factors known to help prevent toxic stress even for those patients with high doses of adversity.

Although there is no standardized method to screen for ACEs, the experience of this article's authors has pointed to the value of universal and routine screening. ACEs screening can be integrated into the standard clinical workflow similar to other pediatric screening tools. The screen is commonly administered by medical staff, reviewed by the medical provider, and the patient is referred to follow-up as appropriate. Various intervention strategies for responding to ACEs are outlined below.

Anticipatory Guidance and Domains of Intervention

Anticipatory guidance

The question remains of what medical providers can do to support the needs of patients and families after they screen for ACEs. A key intervention strategy includes patient/family education and targeted anticipatory guidance. Anticipatory guidance has been shown to be effective in improving child and family functioning in a variety of ways, including violence prevention,[24] sleep, and parent-child interactions.[25,26] Anticipatory guidance is already part of standard pediatric practice, and usually includes education to patients/caregivers about what to expect, or anticipate, over the next few months or years with their child. Recommendations are specific to a child's age at the time of a visit.

Providing anticipatory guidance helps patients/caregivers understand ACEs and toxic stress and be attuned to what types of home, school, or other situations may be causing stress for a child. It gives them information to be able to identify potential symptoms of toxic stress early (eg, difficulty focusing, weight gain/loss, poor control of asthma, poor sleep, anxiety). Anticipatory guidance can also increase a caregiver's understanding of their role as a buffer to children's stress and can help provide tools that caregivers can use to build their children's resilience against adversity.

Anticipatory guidance should always be given with developmentally appropriate knowledge of trauma-informed principles, healing-centered and strengths-based approaches, and cultural humility and implicit bias awareness.[27–30] One of the goals of anticipatory guidance about ACEs should include decreasing blame and shame given that patients and caregivers experiencing trauma-related symptomatology are exhibiting normal physiologic and biological reactions to abnormal, traumatic situations.

Domains of anticipatory guidance for toxic stress
Anticipatory guidance and interventions can focus on the following domains that have specifically been shown to aid in addressing stress and improving some aspects of neuroendocrine and immune function and health outcomes: healthy relationships, sleep, exercise, nutrition, mindfulness, and nature.[31]

Healthy relationships Numerous studies have demonstrated the protective role of caregivers, secure attachment, and their positive influence on children's development.[32–34] Conversely, lack of social integration and/or social support have been shown to be a greater risk factor for mortality in adults than smoking, alcohol consumption, and physical activity levels.[35,36] Just as ACEs have been found to have a dose-dependent negative impact on health, social integration has been found to have a dose-dependent protective effect on health.[37]

It is important to note that parental ACEs and mental health are linked with intergenerational or epigenetic transmission, higher risk of parental stress response dysregulation, lack of coregulation by the caregiver, and lack of modeling self-regulation tools, all leading to greater risk of their children being exposed to adversity in higher doses without a buffer or internal self-regulation skills.[38–41] Safe, stable, and nurturing relationships can break the intergenerational cycle of abuse.[42] A caregiver can modulate the stress-related emotional and physiologic arousal for the child and calm the child's threat response system.

Medical providers should note the nature of the caregiver-child relationship at every visit and offer support when needed. Attention to relational health for both child and caregiver should start in the prenatal period and extend throughout the lifespan. Medical providers can support the caregiver to tend to their own physical and mental health and well-being such that the caregiver can be a buffer to their child. Self-care for caregivers involves managing their own stress levels through healthy relationships, nutritious meals, adequate sleep, physical activity, mindfulness, and tending to their own mental health.

Sleep Reduced sleep duration and poor sleep quality have been linked to many diseases and even death in both adults and children.[43–45]

A child's bedtime routine, reading books, and limiting screen time before bed to promote sleep hygiene are most often part of standard patient education and anticipatory guidance given by medical providers.[46]

However, if there is instability in a household or in the child's environment, this may impact a child's ability to sleep, leading to the need for an additional anticipatory guidance and stress management tools. Medical providers can encourage caregivers to talk with their child about stressors that may be keeping their child awake and remind them about their role in soothing the threat response system. Studies have also looked at meditation as a sleep tool as well as physical activities and found improvement in sleep quality.[47–49] Detailing medications for sleep in the pediatric population is beyond the scope of this article. Generally, behavioral techniques and sleep hygiene education are first-line interventions.[50] Pediatric medical providers can further review the use of medications, such as melatonin in other review articles on sleep.[50,51]

Nutrition The threat response involves activation of the sympathetic nervous system (SNS) and the HPA axis. Generally, SNS activation involves decreasing appetite and gut mobility and metabolizing energy stores to aid in quick escape. Activation of the HPA axis and cortisol release tends to involve longer-term survival strategies, such as increasing desire for high-calorie, high-fat food to increase reserves for the next stressor.[52–54] Thus, depending on the individual, the adversity they experience, and the length of time over which that adversity has occurred, both the SNS and the HPA axis activation can impact weight gain or loss due to stress. Anticipatory guidance on the biology of stress and its impact on weight may help reduce blame and shame surrounding obesity and offer biologically based tools to intervene.

Knowing that stress can lead to craving high-fat, high-energy foods, medical providers can work with caregivers to identify healthy forms of high-fat, high-energy foods, such as nuts, yogurt, fish, and avocados. Knowing that toxic stress can lead to inflammation and a dysregulated immune system, medical providers can offer education promoting anti-inflammatory foods, such as fruits, vegetables, turmeric, and omega-3 fatty acids and discuss avoiding proinflammatory foods, such as fast food and overly processed foods.[55–59] Gut bacteria may impact the stress response and cognitive functioning, and future research may point to specific probiotics as helpful interventions for stress management.[52,55,60]

Food can also be a core component of culture and relationship across the lifespan, including supporting healthy nutrition for pregnant mothers,[53,56,61] breastfeeding practices, and responsive feeding practices,[53,54,57,62] and eating meals together as a family and with community.

Exercise Adult and animal studies show that physical activity improves brain health, including tests of cognitive functioning and neurogenesis and affects endocrine and immune functioning.[55,63–65] Fewer studies have evaluated the impact of physical activity on children's neuroendocrine and immune function. A few studies have shown a positive association between physical activity and academic performance in elementary school-age children and adolescents[65] and a lower risk of respiratory infections in children.[55,58,63,66] Given the comorbidity risk with obesity, exercise may help with weight loss and cardio-pulmonary function, including asthma management improvement.[56,59,64,67] In addition, physical activity may improve other domains of wellness, including sleep and psychological functioning.[49]

Activation of the threat response system is associated with changes in metabolic factors, including insulin and glucose.[43] Children who experience an acute stressor but must sit still in the classroom setting or stay inside at home due to fear of community violence, may not have an outlet to metabolize the extra energy released into their bloodstream. Exercise can help metabolize that energy and regulate the stress response for children and families.[57,60,65,68] Programs that couple physical activity with character development, such as martial arts or mindfulness practices, such as yoga, may lead to more improvements in executive functioning.[58,61,66,69]

Medical providers can discuss the stress-related health benefits of physical activity with caregivers, create treatment plans that include fun physical activities for both the child and their caregiver, and connect families with community resources offering physical activity programs.

Mindfulness Mindfulness and meditation have been defined and evaluated in various ways with varying specificity, making research into their impact on physiology and health complicated.[59,60,62,63,67,68,70,71] A frequently used definition of mindfulness by Kabat-Zinn identifies core components, including nonjudgmental, open-hearted, moment-to-moment awareness, and attention in the present moment.[59,61,62,64,67,69,70,72]

Although limitations in definitions and evaluation techniques exist, research on adults suggests that mindfulness-based interventions, including meditation, yoga,

Tai Chi, and Qi Gong can improve a wide range of social, emotional, behavioral and physiologic outcomes.[47,62–67,70–75]

Studies in children suggest that yoga, mindfulness, and meditation programs may improve symptoms of behavioral mental health.[65–70,73–78] Mindfulness programs may also help foster resilience and decrease parental stress[68,71,76,79] and can be used by providers as potential interventions to manage stress for children and caregivers to improve outcomes. Medical providers can direct patients and families to books with scripts,[69,72,77,80] picture books for younger children,[70,73,78,81] and online tools and applications, including Sesame Workshop.[71,72,74,75,79,80,82,83] In addition, mindfulness practices can enhance other domains of wellness. For example, Progressive Muscle Relaxation and other meditations can help worried children fall asleep.

Nature Ongoing research suggests that spending time in nature may reduce stress and improve health by lowering heart rate, reducing blood pressure, altering cortisol levels, and improving cognitive functioning.[73,76,81,84] Exposure to nature may also help indirectly by increasing physical activity and social contact.[74,77,82,85]

Medical providers can improve access to nature through park prescriptions, partnering with local parks and organizations, and providing families with directions. Park prescriptions were found to increase park visits, decrease perceived stress and loneliness, increase physical activity, decrease cortisol levels, and increase resilience.[75,76,78,79,83,84,86,87]

Overall, when discussing and offering anticipatory guidance and interventions for toxic stress with children and families, a hopeful approach is critical. Although primary care medical providers are not expected to be social workers, psychologists, or psychiatrists, ACEs impact health and are, therefore, within the domain of anticipatory guidance to help mitigate and heal toxic stress. For example, telling patients that all of their tests are normal and that therefore their presenting symptoms are not medical is neglecting the limits of our current scientific knowledge on toxic stress and available testing at nonresearch-based labs. In addition, this type of communication strips the patient of hope and empowerment. Thought changes biology. Research has found that thought alone can lead to changes in the immune response and neuroplastic change.[55,77,80] Avoiding the nocebo effect[78,79,81,82,85,86,88,89] and helping patients and families recognize their own strength in overcoming and healing from ACEs is critical to their success. Providers must maintain a close working relationship with their families, support caregivers to be caring and buffering adults, and offer hope for healing, which can include specific intervention tools on sleep, nutrition, physical activity, mindfulness, and nature.

Resources and Referrals

For children with symptoms of toxic stress dysregulation or higher ACE scores, the medical provider may need to refer the child to additional services and supports. The type of referral will vary depending on variables, such as the prominent presenting issue, financial resources, time bandwidth, and geographic location to services. Integrated behavioral health, including care coordination, psychotherapy, and psychiatry may offer support to medical providers in a busy practice. Pediatric office-based and external interventions are essential to meet the more specific needs of patients.

Several research studies have shown that mental health interventions impact physiologic outcomes. Slopen and colleagues[90] conducted a systematic review of interventions to improve cortisol regulation in children.[80,83,87] They found 18 articles that supported evidence for mental health focused interventions lowering cortisol levels. For example, Carlson and Earls[91] implemented a social and educational enrichment program for children for 13 months and found that the intervention group had lower noontime cortisol compared with controls.[81,84,88,91] In addition, support programs and psychological interventions have been shown to improve health outcomes, such as lowering blood pressure and improving diabetes management.[82,83,85,86,89,90,92,93]

Integrated behavioral health models: These models combine medical and behavioral health services to more fully address the spectrum of problems that patients bring. The goal is to treat both behavioral and physical problems in the most acceptable and effective way to yield the best results for the patient.

Care coordination: The core elements shared among care coordination models include assessment, case management, and referral to social services. Pediatric clinics should highly consider employing non-physician(s) to assist with education and care coordination.

Critical aspects of coordinated care in pediatrics include a tailored, partnership-based approach to the patient's condition and the family's situation, well-defined goals, and a single care coordinator assigned to the family who is in regular contact with them and various health care professionals involved in their care.[84,87,91,94] Patient- and family-centered care coordination can help problem-solve around social determinants of health, including ACEs, and connect families to external resources and referrals.[85,88,92,95]

Psychotherapy: There are a variety of evidence-supported treatments and promising practices that share core principles of culturally competent, trauma-informed therapy that are appropriate for children and families from diverse cultural backgrounds. These may include:

- Child parent psychotherapy[86,89,93,96]
- Parent-child interaction therapy[87,88,90,91,94,95,97,98]
- Trauma-focused cognitive behavioral therapy[89,92,96,99]
- Dialectical behavioral therapy[90,93,97,100]
- Cue-centered therapy[91,94,98,101]
- Eye movement desensitization and reprocessing[92,95,99,102]
- Biofeedback and neurofeedback[93,94,96,97,100,101,103,104]

Psychiatry: Psychiatrists may be a critical part of the integrated health team depending on the severity of the presenting symptoms. It is important to identify psychiatrists who (1) understand the biology and physiology of trauma, (2) recognize developmental trauma disorder,[95,98,102,105] and do not over diagnose or inadvertently misdiagnose children exposed to ACEs with other conditions, such as oppositional defiant disorder or attention deficit hyperactivity disorder, and (3) are cognizant of issues surrounding over medication and polypharmacy use especially with foster youth.[96,99,103,106]

Flora Traub and Renée Boynton-Jarrett[107] offer insightful recommendations to pediatric practices to improve resilience to ACEs, including: (1) train all staff in trauma-informed care, (2) screen risk and protective factors, (3) employ non-physicians to help with screening, education, and care coordination, (4) create a medical home, (5) create an integrated behavioral health program, (6) offer group-based parenting support and education, (7) offer peer-based education, (8) customize health care to the needs of the family, (9) identify local resources, and (10) be aware of barriers to engagement.[97,100,104,107] In addition, the American Academy of Pediatrics offers a Trauma Guide, which includes "Trauma Toolbox for Primary Care,"[108] "Helping Foster and Adoptive Families Cope With Trauma: A Guide for Pediatricians,"[98,101,105,108,109] and additional resources.

SUMMARY

The ACE study demonstrates that adversity is common and impacts a wide range of health outcomes.[1] Increasing research is highlighting the physiologic and biological mechanisms, often encapsulated by the theory of toxic stress, which lead to these behavioral, mental, and physical outcomes.[5,6,18,23]

Because ACEs are a risk factor for health conditions, such as depression, anxiety, asthma, obesity, diabetes, and heart disease, it is incumbent on pediatric medical providers to screen and intervene. Primary care is the ideal setting for ACEs screening because interacting with children and their families at regular intervals can allow patients and providers to develop a trusting relationship and address common misconceptions, which can facilitate the disclosure of ACEs and provides an opportunity for education and continued monitoring. Providers can advance the health and well-being of children and families affected by ACEs by (1) identifying children and families in need through ACEs screening, (2) offering empathetic and science-based anticipatory guidance, including expanded education and interventions related to healthy relationships, sleep, nutrition, physical activity, mindfulness, nature, and mental health, and (3) providing trauma-focused and human-centered resources and referrals when needed.

DISCLOSURE

The authors have nothing to disclose.

REFERENCE

1. Felitti VJ, Anda RF, Nordenberg D, et al. Relationship of childhood abuse and household dysfunction to many of the leading causes of death in adults: the Adverse Childhood Experiences (ACE) Study. Am J Prev Med 1998;14:245–58.
2. Robert Wood Johnson Foundation. The truth about ACEs. Princeton (NJ): Robert Wood Johnson Foundation; 2013.
3. Gilbert R, Widom CS, Browne K, et al. Burden and consequences of child maltreatment in high-income countries. Lancet 2009;373:68–81.
4. Felitti VJ. Adverse childhood experiences and adult health. Acad Pediatr 2009; 9:131–2.
5. Bucci M, Marques SS, Oh D, et al. Toxic stress in children and adolescents. Adv Pediatr 2016;63:403–28.
6. Johnson SB, Riley AW, Granger DA, et al. The science of early life toxic stress for pediatric practice and advocacy. Pediatrics 2013;131:319–27.
7. Kalmakis KA, Chandler GE. Health consequences of adverse childhood experiences: a systematic review. J Am Assoc Nurse Pract 2015. https://doi.org/10.1002/2327-6924.12215.
8. Hughes K, Bellis MA, Hardcastle KA, et al. The effect of multiple adverse childhood experiences on health: a systematic review and meta-analysis. Lancet Public Health 2017;2:e356–66.
9. Oh DL, Jerman P, Silvério Marques S, et al. Systematic review of pediatric health outcomes associated with childhood adversity. BMC Pediatr 2018;18.
10. Burke NJ, Hellman JL, Scott BG, et al. The impact of adverse childhood experiences on an urban pediatric population. Child Abuse Negl 2011;35:408–13.
11. Duke NN, Pettingell SL, McMorris BJ, et al. Adolescent violence perpetration: associations with multiple types of adverse childhood experiences. Pediatrics 2010;125:e778–86.

12. Enlow MB, Egeland B, Blood EA, et al. Interpersonal trauma exposure and cognitive development in children to age 8 years: a longitudinal study. J Epidemiol Community Health 2012;66(11):1005–10.

13. Strathearn L, Gray PH, O'Callaghan MJ, et al. Childhood neglect and cognitive development in extremely low birth weight infants: a prospective study. Pediatrics 2001;108:142–51.

14. Richards M, Wadsworth MEJ. Long term effects of early adversity on cognitive function. Arch Dis Child 2004;89:922–7.

15. Koita K, Long D, Hessler D, et al. Development and implementation of a pediatric adverse childhood experiences (ACEs) and other determinants of health questionnaire in the pediatric medical home: A pilot study. PLoS One 2018; 13:e0208088.

16. Behavioral risk factor surveillance system ACE Data |Violence Prevention|Injury Center|CDC. 2019. Available at: https://www.cdc.gov/violenceprevention/childabuseandneglect/acestudy/ace-brfss.html. Accessed April 18, 2019.

17. Bethell CD, Newacheck P, Hawes E, et al. Adverse childhood experiences: assessing the impact on health and school engagement and the mitigating role of resilience. Health Aff (Millwood) 2014;33:2106–15.

18. Garner AS, Shonkoff JP, Committee on Psychosocial Aspects of Child and Family Health, Committee on Early Childhood, Adoption, and Dependent Care, Section on Developmental and Behavioral Pediatrics. Early childhood adversity, toxic stress, and the role of the pediatrician: translating developmental science into lifelong health. Pediatrics 2012;129:e224–31.

19. American Academy of Pediatrics. The medical home approach to identifying and responding to exposure to trauma 2014. Available at: https://www.aap.org/en-us/Documents/ttb_medicalhomeapproach.pdf https://www.aap.org/en-us/Documents/ttb_medicalhomeapproach.pdf. Accessed June 20, 2019.

20. Franke HA. Toxic stress: effects, prevention and treatment. Children 2014;1: 390–402.

21. Goldstein E, Athale N, Sciolla AF, et al. Patient preferences for discussing childhood trauma in primary care. Perm J 2017;21:16-055.

22. Merrick MT, Leeb RT, Lee RD. Examining the role of safe, stable, and nurturing relationships in the intergenerational continuity of child maltreatment—introduction to the special issue. J Adolesc Health 2013;53:S1–3.

23. Shonkoff JP, Garner AS, Committee on Psychosocial Aspects of Child and Family Health, Committee on Early Childhood, Adoption, and Dependent CareSection on Developmental and Behavioral Pediatrics. The lifelong effects of early childhood adversity and toxic stress. Pediatrics 2011;129:e232.

24. Sege RD, Hatmaker-Flanigan E, Vos ED, et al. Anticipatory guidance and violence prevention: results from family and pediatrician focus groups. Pediatrics 2006;117:455–63.

25. Nelson CS, Wissow LS, Cheng TL. Effectiveness of anticipatory guidance: recent developments. Curr Opin Pediatr 2003;15:630–5.

26. Hsu H-C, Lee S-Y, Lai C-M, et al. Effects of pediatric anticipatory guidance on mothers of young children. West J Nurs Res 2018;40:305–26.

27. Marsac ML, Kassam-Adams N, Hildenbrand AK, et al. Implementing a trauma-informed approach in pediatric health care networks. JAMA Pediatr 2016; 170:70–7.

28. Ginwright S. The future of healing: shifting from trauma informed care to healing centered engagement. Alexandria (VA): Kindship Carers Victoria/Grandparents Victoria; 2018.

29. Boynton-Jarrett R, Flacks J. Strengths-based approaches to screening families for health-related social needs in the healthcare setting. New York: Center For The Study Of Social Policy; 2018.

30. Derrington SF, Paquette E, Johnson KA. Cross-cultural interactions and shared decision-making. Pediatrics 2018;142:S187–92.

31. Harris NB. The deepest well: healing the long-term effects of childhood adversity. Boston (MA): Houghton Mifflin Harcourt; 2018.

32. Blum D. Love at Goon Park: Harry Harlow and the science of affection. New York: Basic Books; 2002.

33. Meaney MJ, Szyf M. Maternal care as a model for experience-dependent chromatin plasticity? Trends Neurosci 2005;28:456–63.

34. Lieberman AF, Padrón E, Horn PV, et al. Angels in the nursery: the intergenerational transmission of benevolent parental influences. Infant Ment Health J 2005; 26:504–20.

35. Holt-Lunstad J, Smith TB, Layton JB. Social relationships and mortality risk: a meta-analytic review. PLoS Med 2010;7:e1000316.

36. Holt-Lunstad J. Why social relationships are important for physical health: a systems approach to understanding and modifying risk and protection. Annu Rev Psychol 2018;69:437–58.

37. Yang YC, Boen C, Gerken K, et al. Social relationships and physiological determinants of longevity across the human life span. Proc Natl Acad Sci 2016;113: 578–83.

38. Lyons-Ruth K, Holmes BM, Sasvari-Szekely M, et al. Serotonin transporter polymorphism and borderline or antisocial traits among low-income young adults. Psychiatr Genet 2007;17:339–43.

39. Schore AN. The right brain is dominant in psychotherapy. Psychotherapy 2014; 51:388–97.

40. Gunnar MR, Donzella B. Social regulation of the cortisol levels in early human development. Psychoneuroendocrinology 2002;27:199–220.

41. Sroufe LA. Attachment and development: a prospective, longitudinal study from birth to adulthood. Attach Hum Dev 2005;7:349–67.

42. Jaffee SR, Bowes L, Ouellet-Morin I, et al. Safe, stable, nurturing relationships break the intergenerational cycle of abuse: a prospective nationally representative cohort of children in the United Kingdom. J Adolesc Health 2013;53:S4–10.

43. McEwen BS. Physiology and neurobiology of stress and adaptation: central role of the brain. Physiol Rev 2007;87:873–904.

44. Itani O, Jike M, Watanabe N, et al. Short sleep duration and health outcomes: a systematic review, meta-analysis, and meta-regression. Sleep Med 2017;32: 246–56.

45. Gallicchio L, Kalesan B. Sleep duration and mortality: a systematic review and meta-analysis. J Sleep Res 2009;18:148–58.

46. Owens JA. The practice of pediatric sleep medicine: results of a community survey. Pediatrics 2001;108:E51.

47. Black DS, O'Reilly GA, Olmstead R, et al. Mindfulness meditation and improvement in sleep quality and daytime impairment among older adults with sleep disturbances: a randomized clinical trial. JAMA Intern Med 2015;175:494–501.

48. Nagendra RPM, Maruthai NMP, Kutty BMMP. Meditation and its regulatory role on sleep. Front Neurol 2012;3:54.

49. Lang C, Brand S, Feldmeth AK, et al. Increased self-reported and objectively assessed physical activity predict sleep quality among adolescents. Physiol Behav 2013;120:46–53.

50. Badin E, Haddad C, Shatkin JP. Insomnia: the sleeping giant of pediatric public health. Curr Psychiatry Rep 2016;18:47.

51. Abdelgadir IS, Gordon MA, Akobeng AK. Melatonin for the management of sleep problems in children with neurodevelopmental disorders: a systematic review and meta-analysis. Arch Dis Child 2018;103:1155–62.

52. Romeo J, Warnberg J, Gómez-Martínez S, et al. Neuroimmunomodulation by nutrition in stress situations. Neuroimmunomodulation 2008;15:165–9.

53. Wardle J, Gibson EL. Chapter 55 - diet and stress: interactions with emotions and behavior. In: Fink G, editor. Stress: concepts, cognition, emotion, and behavior. Cambridge (MA): Academic Press; 2016. p. 435–43. https://doi.org/10.1016/B978-0-12-800951-2.00058-3.

54. Sims R, Gordon S, Garcia W, et al. Perceived stress and eating behaviors in a community-based sample of African Americans. Eat Behav 2008;9:137–42.

55. Shaffer J. Neuroplasticity and clinical practice: building brain power for health. Front Psychol 2016;7:1118.

56. Aubry AV, Khandaker H, Ravenelle R, et al. A diet enriched with curcumin promotes resilience to chronic social defeat stress. Neuropsychopharmacology 2019;44:733.

57. James A, Abramson M. Fast food and asthma and allergy: be afried, be deeply afried? Respirology 2018;23:881–2.

58. Kiecolt-Glaser JK, Glaser R, Christian LM. Omega-3 fatty acids and stress-induced immune dysregulation: implications for wound healing. Mil Med 2014; 179:129–33.

59. Holt EM, Steffen LM, Moran A, et al. Fruit and vegetable consumption and its relation to markers of inflammation and oxidative stress in adolescents. J Am Diet Assoc 2009;109:414–21.

60. Dinan TG, Cryan JF. Regulation of the stress response by the gut microbiota: Implications for psychoneuroendocrinology. Psychoneuroendocrinology 2012;37: 1369–78.

61. Vohr BR, Davis EP, Wanke CA, et al. Neurodevelopment: the impact of nutrition and inflammation during preconception and pregnancy in low-resource settings. Pediatrics 2017;139:S38–49.

62. Yousafzai AK, Rasheed MA, Bhutta ZA. Annual research review: improved nutrition–pathway to resilience. J Child Psychol Psychiatry 2013;54:367–77.

63. Diamond MC. Response of the brain to enrichment. An Acad Bras Ciênc 2001; 73:211–20.

64. Russell VA, Zigmond MJ, Dimatelis JJ, et al. The interaction between stress and exercise, and its impact on brain function. Metab Brain Dis 2014;29:255–60.

65. Voss MW, Vivar C, Kramer AF, et al. Bridging animal and human models of exercise-induced brain plasticity. Trends Cogn Sci 2013;17:525–44.

66. Jedrychowski W, Maugeri U, Flak E, et al. Cohort study on low physical activity level and recurrent acute respiratory infections in schoolchildren. Cent Eur J Public Health 2001;9:126–9.

67. Lucas JA, Moonie S, Hogan MB, et al. Efficacy of an exercise intervention among children with comorbid asthma and obesity. Public Health 2018;159: 123–8.

68. Sylow L, Kleinert M, Richter EA, et al. Exercise-stimulated glucose uptake - regulation and implications for glycaemic control. Nat Rev Endocrinol 2017; 13:133–48.

69. Diamond A. Effects of physical exercise on executive functions: going beyond simply moving to moving with thought. Ann Sports Med Res 2015;2:1011.

70. Van Dam NT, van Vugt MK, Vago DR, et al. Mind the hype: a critical evaluation and prescriptive agenda for research on mindfulness and meditation. Perspect Psychol Sci 2018;13:36–61.

71. Nash JD, Newberg A. Toward a unifying taxonomy and definition for meditation. Front Psychol 2013;4.

72. Kabat-Zinn J. Mindfulness meditation: health benefits of an ancient Buddhist practice. In: Goleman D, Gurin J, editors. Mind/Body Medicine. Washington, DC: Consumer Reports Books. American Psychological Association; 1993. p. 144–56.

73. Black DS, Semple RJ, Pokhrel P, et al. Component processes of executive function—mindfulness, self-control, and working memory—and their relationships with mental and behavioral health. Mindfulness 2011;2:179–85.

74. Roemer L, Lee JK, Salters-Pedneault K, et al. Mindfulness and emotion regulation difficulties in generalized anxiety disorder: preliminary evidence for independent and overlapping contributions. Behav Ther 2009;40:142–54.

75. Tolahunase MR, Sagar R, Faiq M, et al. Yoga- and meditation-based lifestyle intervention increases neuroplasticity and reduces severity of major depressive disorder: a randomized controlled trial. Restor Neurol Neurosci 2018;36:423–42.

76. Chimiklis A, Dahl V, Spears AP, et al. Yoga, mindfulness, and meditation interventions for youth with ADHD: systematic review and meta-analysis. J Child Fam Stud 2018;27:3155–68.

77. Kallapiran K, Koo S, Kirubakaran R, et al. Review: effectiveness of mindfulness in improving mental health symptoms of children and adolescents: a meta-analysis. Child Adolesc Ment Health 2015;20:182–94.

78. Dunning DL, Griffiths K, Kuyken W, et al. Research review: the effects of mindfulness-based interventions on cognition and mental health in children and adolescents - a meta-analysis of randomized controlled trials. J Child Psychol Psychiatry 2019;60:244–58.

79. Bethell C, Gombojav N, Solloway M, et al. Adverse childhood experiences, resilience and mindfulness-based approaches: common denominator issues for children with emotional, mental, or behavioral problems. Child Adolesc Psychiatr Clin N Am 2016;25:139–56.

80. Snel E. Sitting still like a frog: mindfulness exercises for kids (and their parents). Boulder (CO): Shambhala Publications; 2013.

81. MacLean KL. Moody cow meditates. New York: Simon and Schuster; 2009.

82. Weekly T, Walker N, Beck J, et al. A review of apps for calming, relaxation, and mindfulness interventions for pediatric palliative care patients. Children 2018; 5:16.

83. Oades-Sese GV, Cohen D, Allen JWP, et al. Building resilience in young children the sesame street way. In: Prince-Embury S, Saklofske DH, editors. Resilience interventions for youth in diverse populations. New York: Springer; 2014. p. 181–201. https://doi.org/10.1007/978-1-4939-0542-3_9.

84. Kondo MC, Jacoby SF, South EC. Does spending time outdoors reduce stress? A review of real-time stress response to outdoor environments. Health Place 2018;51:136–50.

85. Kondo MC, Fluehr JM, McKeon T, et al. Urban green space and its impact on human health. Int J Environ Res Public Health 2018;15 [pii:E445].

86. Razani N, Morshed S, Kohn MA, et al. Effect of park prescriptions with and without group visits to parks on stress reduction in low-income parents: SHINE randomized trial. PLoS One 2018;13:e0192921.

87. Razani N, Niknam K, Wells NM, et al. Clinic and park partnerships for childhood resilience: a prospective study of park prescriptions. Health Place 2019;57: 179–85.

88. Bingel U. Avoiding nocebo effects to optimize treatment outcome. JAMA 2014; 312:693–4.

89. Colloca L, Finniss D. Nocebo effects, patient-clinician communication, and therapeutic outcomes. JAMA 2012;307:567–8.

90. Slopen N, McLaughlin KA, Shonkoff JP. Interventions to improve cortisol regulation in children: a systematic review. Pediatrics 2014;133:312–26.

91. Carlson M, Earls F. Psychological and neuroendocrinological sequelae of early social deprivation in institutionalized children in Romania. Ann N Y Acad Sci 1997;807:419–28.

92. Harkness E, Macdonald W, Valderas J, et al. Identifying psychosocial interventions that improve both physical and mental health in patients with diabetes: a systematic review and meta-analysis. Diabetes Care 2010;33:926–30.

93. Ahmadpanah M, Paghale SJ, Bakhtyari A, et al. Effects of psychotherapy in combination with pharmacotherapy, when compared to pharmacotherapy only on blood pressure, depression, and anxiety in female patients with hypertension. J Health Psychol 2016;21:1216–27.

94. Moreno MA. Pediatric care coordination. JAMA Pediatr 2019;173:112.

95. Kuo DZ, McAllister JW, Rossignol L, et al. Care coordination for children with medical complexity: whose care is it, anyway? Pediatrics 2018;141:S224–32.

96. Lieberman AF, Ippen CG, Hernandez Dimmler M. Assessing and treating youth exposed to traumatic stress. Washington, DC: American Psychiatric Pub; 2018.

97. Funderburk BW, Eyberg S. Parent–child interaction therapy. In: History of psychotherapy: continuity and change. 2nd edition. Washington, DC: American Psychological Association; 2011. p. 415–20. https://doi.org/10.1037/12353-021.

98. Vanderzee KL, Sigel BA, Pemberton JR, et al. Treatments for early childhood trauma: decision considerations for clinicians. J Child Adolesc Trauma 2018. https://doi.org/10.1007/s40653-018-0244-6.

99. Cohen JA, Mannarino AP, Deblinger E. Treating trauma and traumatic grief in children and adolescents. 2nd edition. New York: Guilford Publications; 2016.

100. Steil R, Dittmann C, Müller-Engelmann M, et al. Dialectical behaviour therapy for posttraumatic stress disorder related to childhood sexual abuse: a pilot study in an outpatient treatment setting. Eur J Psychotraumatol 2018;9:1423832.

101. Carrion VG, Kletter H, Weems CF, et al. Cue-centered treatment for youth exposed to interpersonal violence: a randomized controlled trial. J Trauma Stress 2013;26:654–62.

102. Shapiro F, Maxfield L. Eye movement desensitization and reprocessing (EMDR): information processing in the treatment of trauma. J Clin Psychol 2002;58: 933–46.

103. Fisher SF. Neurofeedback in the treatment of developmental trauma: calming the fear-driven brain. New York: W. W. Norton & Company; 2014.

104. Fisher SF, Lanius RA, Frewen PA. EEG neurofeedback as adjunct to psychotherapy for complex developmental trauma-related disorders: case study and treatment rationale. Traumatology 2016;22:255–60.

105. van der Kolk BA. The body keeps score: approaches to the psychobiology of posttraumatic stress disorder. In: Traumatic stress: the effects of overwhelming experience on mind, body, and society. New York: Guilford Press; 1996. p. 214–41.

106. Naylor MW, Davidson CV, Ortega-Piron DJ, et al. Psychotropic medication management for youth in state care: consent, oversight, and policy considerations. Child Welfare 2007;86:175–92.

107. Traub F, Boynton-Jarrett R. Modifiable resilience factors to childhood adversity for clinical pediatric practice. Pediatrics 2017;139:e20162569.

108. American Academy of Pediatrics. Helping foster and adoptive families cope with trauma: a guide for pediatricians. Itasca (IL): American Academy Of Pediatrics; 2016.

109. American Academy of Pediatrics. Helping foster and adoptive families cope with trauma. Itasca (IL): American Academy Of Pediatrics; 2013.

Twenty Questions (and Answers) About Media Violence and Cyberbullying

Marjorie Hogan, MD[a],*, Victor Strasburger, MD[b]

KEYWORDS

- Media violence • Video game violence • Cyberbullying

KEY POINTS

- A robust body of research finds an association between violence on television and in movies and real-life childhood and adolescent aggression, both short and long term.
- Exposure to violent video games may lead to desensitization to violence, acceptance of violence as a response to conflict, and aggressive behavior in some children and teens.
- Cyberbullying, with parallels to face-to-face bullying, is an emerging form of aggression occurring in every major social media platform.
- Parents, schools, pediatricians and other health care providers, and the government must be involved in understanding and mitigating the potential harm posed by media violence and cyberbullying.

INTRODUCTION

Media violence and its impact on young viewers has raised alarms for pediatricians and other professionals for decades, leading to many official statements reviewing the research and issuing recommendations for families. Naturally, early studies and concerns reflected violent images and messages on television (TV) only (Newt Minnow's[1] "vast wasteland") (**Fig. 1**). Recommendations included limiting time watching TV, choosing programs wisely, and encouraging parents to coview with children. A plethora of studies (cross-sectional, laboratory, observational, longitudinal, and meta-analyses) has documented a risk for aggressive thoughts, beliefs, attitudes, and behaviors in some children and teens.[2–7]

Over the next many years, similar concerns arose with violent depictions in popular movies, and then with violent video games with their increasing popularity. Although

[a] Department of Pediatrics, University of Minnesota, Hennepin County Medical Center, 701 Park Avenue, Green 7, Minneapolis, MN 55415, USA; [b] University of New Mexico School of Medicine, Albuquerque, NM, USA
* Corresponding author.
E-mail address: hogan003@umn.edu

Pediatr Clin N Am 67 (2020) 275–291
https://doi.org/10.1016/j.pcl.2019.12.002
pediatric.theclinics.com

"Contrary to the popular view our studies show that it is real life that contributes to violence on television."

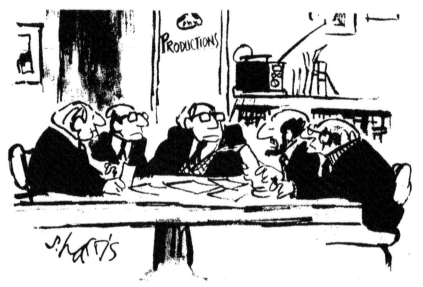

Fig. 1. The impact of media violence is real. (Copyright © Sidney Harris. *ScienceCartoonsPlus.com*.)

some disagreement about the effect of violent video games persists among researchers, professionals, and the public, a preponderance of data suggests that exposure to violence in video games, like media violence in TV and movies, is one risk factor for aggressive behavior in real life[8–10] (see **Fig. 1**).

Aggression is defined as any action intended to cause harm to another who is motivated to avoid harm; violence is an extreme form of aggression intended to cause severe physical harm, such as injury or death. All violent acts are aggressive, whereas not all aggressive acts are violent.[2] Relational aggression includes acts that are intended to harm others emotionally rather than physically, such as gossip, insults, and cyberbullying.

ARE VIOLENT VIDEO GAMES RESPONSIBLE FOR MASS SHOOTINGS AND SCHOOL SHOOTINGS?

This has become the major question in the past decade given the number of mass shootings and school shootings. Such tragedies are difficult to comprehend, and so people go searching for easy answers. There are none. There will never be a study that directly links school and mass shootings to media violence because, as difficult as it is to believe, such shootings are still rare. It would take a sample population of millions of people to try to establish a cause-and-effect link.

Notwithstanding, perpetrators in the many deadly mass shootings over the 20 years since Columbine often played violent video games, and some even practiced shooting skills on the small screen. The Norway killer of 77 people practiced on first-person shooter video games, as did the Beltway killer. Dylan Kliebold and Eric Harris (Columbine), Adam Lanza (Newtown), and Nikolas Cruz (Parkland) were all enamored of first-person shooter games.[10] Even so, large violent events such as Columbine, Sandy Hook, the Pulse nightclub, the high school in Parkland, and many more happen for a multitude of reasons, some unique to each event, others revealing common threads. One theory is that there are 5 factors involved in teens' mass shootings, and the more factors at play, the greater the likelihood of a disaster: (1) social isolation; (2) a history of being bullied or abused; (3) mental illness; (4) heavy exposure to first-person shooter video games; and (5) easy access to guns.[10]

IS THERE A GOOD THEORY TO EXPLAIN THE CONNECTION BETWEEN MEDIA VIOLENCE AND REAL-LIFE VIOLENCE?

In general, media researchers and psychologists acknowledge that aggression and real-life violence are multifactorial in nature. Media violence is only 1 contributory factor to real-life violence. The general aggression model (GAM) is a useful, common-sense theory that considers aggressive behavior to be an interplay of various complex processes unique to each individual.[11,12] GAM is a "dynamic theory that is concerned with how life experiences — in combination with biological and individual differences — create knowledge structures that are the basis of personality, and how these knowledge structures influence affect, cognition, and arousal in specific social encounters to influence the likelihood of aggressive or nonaggressive behavior."[12] The theory posits that violent media exposure may incite aggressive behavior in a given situation in the short term: scripts for response to aggressive situations (seen in media portrayals) then may be retrieved, individuals may mimic aggressive behavior, or media violence may stimulate physiologic arousal.[12] Long-term increases in aggressive attitudes and behavior are explained by observational learning, desensitization to violence, and fear (a belief that the world is a mean and scary place[7,13]) (**Fig. 2**).

In 2018, the International Society for Research on Aggression (ISRA) reviewed the antecedents of youth violence and the research literature.[14] Investigators categorized risk factors into 2 groups: personal and environmental. Personal (individual) risk factors included male gender, aggressive behavior in childhood, and certain personality traits, whereas environmental factors included access to guns, social isolation, family discord or violence, school opportunities, substance use, and exposure to media violence.[12] Significantly, "many risk factors such as gender, parental criminality, traumatic family experiences, and exposure to media violence are shared by individuals who will never become violent."[14] Some risk factors are immutable (eg, gender and history of family violence) but others, notably access to guns and exposure to violent media, are amenable to change. Even some personality traits may be altered through interventions for anger management, skill building, and enhancing empathy. ISRA suggested that parents and other adults can work to build supportive communities and services for at-risk youth.[14]

HOW GOOD IS THE RESEARCH?

No research is perfect, and social science research is particularly fraught with obstacles and differing interpretations.[15] Teasing out specific influences on human behavior is virtually a mission impossible. However, the research is clear on this subject and has been for a long time; so long that there is very little ongoing research on the impact of

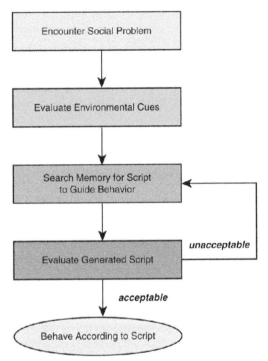

Fig. 2. How scripts contribute to aggressive behavior. (*From*: Strasburger VC, Wilson BJ, Jordan AB. *Children, Adolescents, and the Media*, 3rd ed. Los Angeles: Sage, 2014, reprinted with permission.)

TV or movie violence, only video game violence. The preponderance of peer-reviewed studies over the past 3 to 4 decades confirms that exposure to violent images and messages in various media is associated with aggressive attitudes and behavior in some children and teens. Of course, there are skeptics and deniers, just as there are deniers of climate change, the moon landing, and the Holocaust. The conclusion is that the association between media violence and aggression is stronger than the effect of several very commonly accepted public health risks (**Fig. 3**).

This scientific research uses a range of study designs, including laboratory, correlational, observational, and longitudinal studies, and meta-analyses, and shows (with some exceptions) that exposure to media violence can contribute to aggressive behavior and other harmful outcomes, including decrease in empathy and prosocial behavior. A prominent media researcher, Dr Douglas Gentile, specifically reviewing the 2015 American Psychological Association (APA) Task Force on Violent Media resolution and a 2018 meta-analysis of 24 studies published in the *Proceedings of the National Academy of Science*, stated: "media violence is one risk factor for aggression. It's not the biggest, it's also not the smallest, but it's worth paying attention to"[16–18] (**Box 1**).

Laboratory studies have consistently found exposure to violent media to be associated in the short-term with "increased aggressive thoughts, angry feelings, physiological arousal, hostile appraisals, aggressive behavior, and desensitization to violence"[2] as well as a decrease in "prosocial behavior and empathy."[2]

One of the most powerful ways of showing a connection between exposure to variable and subsequent outcomes is a longitudinal correlational study. Among the best

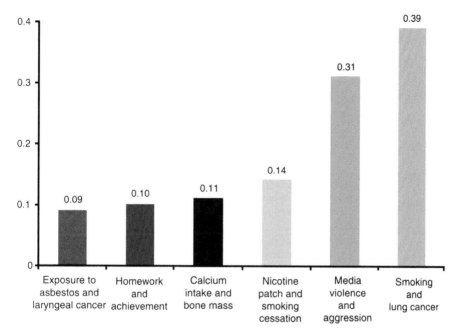

Fig. 3. How media violence fits into commonly accepted public health risks. (*From*: Strasburger VC, Wilson BJ, Jordan AB. Children, Adolescents, and the Media, 3rd ed. Los Angeles: Sage, 2014, reprinted with permission.)

have been the studies of Huesmann and Eron: they examined the TV violence viewing habits of 427 third-grade children and their adult aggressive behavior 15 years later, finding a positive prediction for both genders. This finding suggested that "both males and females from all social strata and all levels of initial aggressiveness are placed at increased risk for the development of adult aggressive and violent behavior when they view a high and steady diet of violent TV shows in early childhood."[7,19,20] In the same study, there was not a relationship between aggressive behavior in childhood and choosing to view TV violence at age 19 years (**Fig. 4**).[19] Huesman and colleagues[20] found the same results for children in Finland and other countries as well: "For girls in the United States and boys in both countries, TV violence viewing was significantly related to concurrent aggression and significantly predicted future changes in aggression. The strength of the relation depended as much on the frequency with which violence was viewed as on the extent of the violence." A follow up study of the same cohort found that "criminal behavior at age 30 … was predicted by their age 8 violence viewing."[6] Even more compelling, a 15-year longitudinal study followed children in elementary school, finding that "boys and girls who watched more TV violence in early childhood were significantly more aggressive young adults, independent of how aggressive they had been during childhood," [19] even controlling for different parenting styles, intelligence measures, and social class.

Experts identify several reasons for the association between screen and real-life aggression and violence. First, children learn by imitation, whether positive or harmful behaviors, whether from real people or characters on a screen. This idea is the social learning theory, first espoused by Bandura in 1960.[21,22] When children see and hear violent images and messages on a screen, they are learning powerful lessons, depending on the depiction. If characters are "good guys," use violence, and are

Box 1
A brief history of media violence research and responses

1933: Publication of the Payne Fund Studies, the first significant study on the effects of media on youth.

1954: US Senate holds hearings on whether media violence contributes to juvenile delinquency.

1960s: Classic experimental studies on media violence by Albert Bandura at Stanford using Bobo the Clown.

1972: US Surgeon General issues a report on media violence; publication in *American Psychologist* of the first set of data from Eron and Huesmann's longitudinal study of 8-year-olds.

1982: Publication of a 10-volume, comprehensive report on children and media by the National Institute of Mental Health. 1984 to 1986: Huesmann and colleagues report on the results of their 22-year longitudinal study of 8-year-olds and media violence, which found a highly significant correlation between viewing TV violence in the third grade and aggressive behavior 10 and 22 years later.

1992: A review by the APA estimates that the average American child or teenager sees 10,000 murders, rapes, and aggravated assaults per year on TV alone.

1993: After the release of Death Race, an ultraviolent video game in which hit-and-run drivers obliterate wheelchair-bound octogenarians, the US Senate holds hearings on violent video games, leading to the development of a video game rating system.

1994: Comstock and Paik publish a meta-analysis of more than 215 empirical studies, which found large effect sizes ($r = 0.31$, which means that media violence may be responsible for at least 10% of real-life violence).

1998: The largest study ever undertaken of American TV, the National Television Violence Study (NTVS), examines nearly 10,000 hours of TV and finds that 60% of all programs contain violence and that children's programming is more violent than adults' programming.

2000: The American Academy of Pediatrics (AAP) is joined by the American Medical Association, the American Academy of Child and Adolescent Psychiatry, and the APA in issuing an unprecedented joint statement on the effect of entertainment violence on children in testimony before Congress.

2001: US Surgeon General issues a report on youth violence and cites media violence as a contributing factor.

2003: A panel of media-violence experts convened by the National Institute of Mental Health, at the request of the US Surgeon General, publishes its comprehensive report on the effects of media violence on youth, which reveals media violence to be a significant causal factor in aggression and violence.

2007: The Federal Communications Commission (FCC) releases its report on violent TV programming and its effects on children and agrees with the Surgeon General that there is strong evidence that exposure to media violence can increase aggressive behavior in children.

2012: The ISRA issues a report from its Media Violence Commission.

2016: AAP policy statement issued on virtual violence.

Adapted from Strasburger VC. Twenty questions about media violence and its effect on adolescents. *Adolesc Med: State of the Art Reviews*. 2014; 25(2):473–488; with permission.

rewarded for their violence, children learn that violence is justified and a morally sound and effective way to confront problems. They may also be learning that violence should be the first response to a conflict, rather than negotiation or cooperation. Attractive characters, and those relatable to children, whether people, animals, or fantasy figures, are more likely to be imitated. Children also learn scripts for behavior from

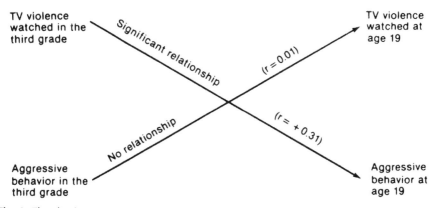

Fig. 4. The classic Huesmann and Eron longitudinal study. (*From*: Strasburger VC, Wilson BJ, Jordan AB. Children, Adolescents, and the Media, third ed, Los Angeles: Sage, 2014; with permission.)

the media (eg, what to do in a given situation, how to respond, whether to let someone get away with an insult). Scripts are stored and can be retrieved when a conflict arises. A key question is, do stored scripts encourage the child to negotiate and compromise when conflicts arise, or is a resort to aggression more likely to be used?

A recent large study across 7 countries found exposure to violent media associated with aggressive behavior positively and significantly, even when other individual risk factors were considered.[11] A 2018 study examined 24 studies and found consistent effects in longitudinal studies that violent video game play and physical aggression are associated over time.[18] As the author states: "A lot of people ask, do these games really cause these kids to behave aggressively? I would say that is one possibility … The other possibility is that it's a really bad sign. If your kids are playing these games, either these games are having a warping effect on right and wrong or they have a warped sense of right or wrong and that's why they are attracted to these games. Either way you should be concerned about it."[23]

Desensitization to violence is another negative outcome of viewing or playing violent media (**Fig. 5**). Studies have shown decreased evidence of physiologic arousal to violent depictions over time. The question of whether physiologic numbing translates into a callousness or indifference to violence is crucial.[3] If so, the implications for society loom large; so, for example, do people feel empathy for those affected? Everyone may be affected to some degree: the so-called third-person effect suggests that people typically think that others may be affected by violence, but they themselves are immune[24] (see **Fig. 5**).

Exposure to violence also can lead to fear in children, the so-called mean and scary world effect. If a child views repeated portrayals of violence on screen, understanding that young children in particular may have some blurring of the media world and the real world, fearing for their own safety and well-being is real. Viewers also incorporate harmful stereotypes from media, possibly leading to increased risk of victimization for those groups.[13,25] More recently, experts studied children's physiologic responses to violent video game exposure, finding that cortisol levels and cardiovascular arousal increased as well as the accessibility of aggressive thoughts. So children playing a violent video game can activate their sympathetic nervous systems and fight-or-flight responses. "Coupled with an increased activation of aggression-related thoughts from violent video game exposure,"[26] the fight-or-flight response may lead to a higher risk of an aggressive act, if provoked.

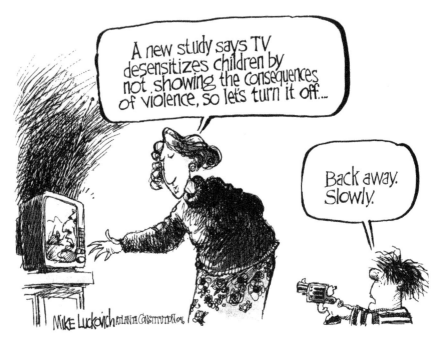

Fig. 5. The densensitization effect. (By permission of Mike Luckovich and Creators Syndicate, Inc.)

ARE VIOLENT VIDEO GAMES MORE HARMFUL THAN VIOLENT TELEVISION SHOWS OR MOVIES?

The potential harm from video game violence parallels what is known about TV violence. Violence that is rewarded, violence perpetrated from a relatable character, and scripts for response to threat or conflict all reinforce aggressive attitudes and behavior, no matter the platform. However, video games (whether on a dedicated platform, a phone, or on a computer) feature intrinsic enticements that provide rewards for successful violence, such as moving to a new level, chances to play in a competitive mode with others, and active participation rather than passive viewing. The child or teenager is now the aggressor. Video games also provide reinforcement through repetition of sequences, imprinting scripts more indelibly. The player may also identify more closely with the aggressor in games, and video games can create a realistic, hostile virtual reality.[27,28]

DOES CYBERBULLYING QUALIFY AS MEDIA VIOLENCE?

Cyberbullying occurs in every major social media platform and represents the new technological form of bullying. A Pew survey in 2018 found that nearly 60% of teens, of both genders, experienced cyberbullying in one of many forms: name calling, rumor spreading, sexting, feeling stalked (constantly being asked intrusive questions), physical threats.[29] Most teens who experience cyberbullying also experience in-person bullying. Outcomes for victims (and abusers) run the gamut from depression, anxiety, and risk of suicide to school dysfunction. New research from a long-term British study showed that "children who are bullied – and especially those who are frequently bullied – continue to be at risk for a wide range of poor social, health, and economic outcomes NEARLY FOUR DECADES after exposure."[30]

Many experts think that cyberbullying is even more dangerous than in-person bullying because (1) the bully is unknown; (2) the bullying remains in cyberspace forever; and (3) the child or teenager's bedroom is no longer a safe haven, especially when there is technology present in the bedroom. Teens think that cyberbullying is a major problem and that antibullying efforts are not currently successful. Most parents also consider cyberbullying and sexting to be significant risks for their teens.[29]

WHY IS THERE STILL A CONTROVERSY?

Although the bulk of scientific research over the decades confirms the association between media violence and harmful outcomes in children and teens, there is not complete consensus.[15] In 2017, the multidisciplinary Work Group on Media Violence and Violent Video Games reviewed 60 years of relevant research, including longitudinal studies and meta-analyses, and found "compelling evidence of short-term harmful effects, as well as evidence of long-term harmful effects."[2] The work group also made the important point that, if media exposure can lead to beneficial outcomes, it follows that exposure to violent images and message can lead to harm. Similarly, Hollywood routinely points to its finest products as inspiring and ennobling; for example, consider recent Academy Award–winning pictures such as 12 Years a Slave, Green Book, and The Shape of Water and older films such as Schindler's List and Saving Private Ryan. However, if great pictures have positive effects, it stands to reason that not-so-great violent films may have negative effects. Researchers who deny substantive harmful impact of violent video games may be losing sight of the prevailing view that exposure to media violence is but 1 risk factor for real-life aggression and violence; it is perhaps not even the most salient risk factor, but it is one that is readily remediable.

IS EVERYONE AFFECTED THE SAME?

Not every smoker develops lung cancer and, similarly, not every child playing violent video games perpetrates violence. Media violence is not the sole, or even the most powerful, antecedent cause of societal violence. Many individual, familial, and societal factors have greater impact on real-life violence. However, unlike exposure to violent media, many of these greater factors are irremediable.

As discussed previously, the GAM offers a complex biosocial-cognitive relationship to understand aggressive behavior on an individual basis: attitudes and behavior evolve with life experiences and are influenced by biological, familial, cultural, and social differences.[11,12]

Children and teens (and also adults) bring their own unique strengths and frailties to the media experience. Those living in homes or neighborhoods rife with guns and violence are likely more susceptible to guns and violence on screens, virtual reality echoing real life.[11,31] Personality traits, levels of resilience, and previous observations about an approach to conflict result in different reactions, both in the short and long term, to playing violent video games. However, just as a long life of daily smoking is more likely to lead to a person's cancer or chronic obstructive pulmonary disease diagnosis, frequent, heavy, repetitive exposure to violent scenes in media may lead to changes in attitude and behavior in the longer term.

CAN MEDIA VIOLENCE EVER BE CATHARTIC?

Some have claimed (without evidence) that, by watching or playing violent media, aggression can be "purged." This theory, first advanced by Aristotle in his Poetics, has never been substantiated by research.[3]

WHY CAN HOLLYWOOD NOT CHANGE?

Well, follow the money. Video games, especially the popular violent games of the day (Call of Duty, Resident Evil, Mortal Combat, and so forth) are big money makers. A violent video game is defined as showing images of intentional harm to another. In 2018, the global video game industry generated nearly $135 billion, an increase of more than 10% from 2017.[32] Americans spent more than $43 billion on video games in 2018, an major increase from $36 billion the previous year.[32,33]

As people have become increasingly desensitized, Hollywood has increased the violence in movies to entice more eyes to theaters and screens. A 2013 study examined the popular James Bond franchise. In a review of 22 Bond films spanning nearly 50 years, the number of violent episodes doubled from 1962 to 2008, and the amount of lethal violence tripled (**Fig. 6**). These portrayals of violence were severe, not trivial, supporting the investigators' hypothesis that movies, in general, have become more violent. In spite of this, the Bond films are rated PG (parental guidance) or PG-13. Implications for movies with an R (restricted) rating, frequently seen by youth, are potentially even more serious[34] (see **Fig. 6**).

IS WITNESSING REAL-LIFE VIOLENCE MORE HARMFUL?

Yes. For both victims and witnesses of violence in childhood, studies show association of such exposure with subsequent trauma symptoms, including behavioral, learning, or emotional difficulties.[35–37] However, this does not diminish the potential harm of viewing violent programs or playing violent games, especially for children and adolescents who live in dangerous homes or neighborhoods. When media violence reflects risks and experiences in real life, the impact logically may be increased.

WHAT CAN PARENTS DO?

Parents can and should play the major role in mitigating the harmful effects of media in their children's lives, as well as maximizing the benefits of positive, prosocial media. For decades, the American Academy of Pediatrics (AAP) has offered helpful advice to parents, focusing on limiting time spent with media, making wise media choices, avoiding media in bedrooms and at the dinner table, and coviewing programs and games. For these recommendations to be successful, the conversation must start in early childhood and continue through adolescence. Parents can and should set

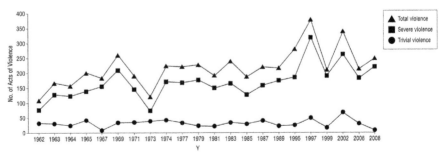

Fig. 6. Increased violence over 4 decades in James Bond movies. (*From* McAnally HM, Robertson LA, Strasburger VC, et al. Bond, James Bond: a review of 46 years of violence in films. *JAMA Pediatr.* 2013 Feb;167(2):195-6. https://doi.org/10.1001/jamapediatrics. 2013.437; with permission.)

appropriate limits on media use in the home and be positive media role models. The AAP's Family Media Use Plan can be accessed online and used by each individual family for their own needs and priorities. Looking at managing media use in the home is analogous to healthy eating: parents need to establish and maintain a healthy media diet.[38,39]

Parents of teens encounter special challenges around media use. Balancing the privacy so coveted and necessary for teens with their safety is a difficult task. Awareness of the common practice of cyberbullying (under the main heading of aggression, if not relational aggression) demands that parents be involved in their teens' media lives, keeping the lines of communication open and being honest about online risks. A survey of teens found that, in general, they appreciate the efforts of their parents in addressing cyberbullying.[29,40,41] The Web sites of Stop the Bullying and the Cyberbullying Research Center offer resources for teens and parents in combatting this common problem.

WHAT CAN CLINICIANS DO?

Pediatricians and other health care providers should support and encourage parents to help their children navigate the media minefield from early childhood. In addition, because the media can affect virtually every area that physicians (and parents) are concerned about (eg, aggression, sex, substance use, obesity, eating disorders, depression, suicide, sleep, and school performance), clinicians must take on this challenge as well. Two salient questions are (1) how many hours daily do the children spend with screens? (2) Is there a TV or Internet connection in the bedroom? As clinicians assess their patients' mental health and social-emotional well-being, they should also ask clear questions about feeling safe at home and school and directly about cyberbullying or in-person bullying.

WHAT CAN SCHOOLS DO?

Now often relying on technology for teaching and homework, schools are pivotal in encouraging healthy media use habits. As part of any health unit, teachers can highlight the association with media, including healthy eating, substance use, sexuality, and safety. This approach constitutes media literacy, and it may represent the new fourth "R" besides reading, writing, and arithmetic. Schools can also encourage students to use technology in creative, positive ways, such as creating apps, videos, and blogs.

Some schools are using social media monitoring systems that use algorithms or keywords to identify potentially troubling posts on public social media, including Twitter and other platforms.[42,43] These new services tout their ability to "help schools prevent everything from sexting and bullying to mass shootings."[44] Although understandably appealing to school administrators and parents, such monitoring systems raise concerns about invasion of adolescents' privacy and the possibility of posts being mistaken or overinterpreted.

WHAT CAN THE GOVERNMENT DO?

Censorship is never the answer to concerns about media content, specifically about violent media. However, the government could and should facilitate research about the short-term and long-term outcomes of violent media exposure for children and teens. The government could easily fund a study section on children and media within the National Institute of Child Health and Human Development (NICHD), elsewhere in the National Institutes of Health (NIH), or within the Centers for Disease Control and Prevention (CDC). Ongoing federal funding (and a home within the government's research agencies) is desperately needed for research on children, adolescents, and the media.

The Children and Media Research Advancement Act (CAMRA Act) was introduced in the US Senate in July 2018 and requires the NIH to fund $40 million of research regarding the effects of media on infants, children, and adolescents. Such research would examine the impact of media (eg, social media, TV, video games) on cognitive, physical, and social-emotional development. The bill is currently moving through the legislative process, but its fate is unknown at this time.[45]

In addition, the US government has a clear responsibility to research and regulate the use of guns. Both Australia and New Zealand moved quickly to ban assault weapons and passed tough gun laws in the immediate aftermath of mass shootings in 2001 and 2019, respectively. Mass shootings in the United States, which have occurred with increasing frequency in the past 2 decades, have elicited no action in Congress, in large part because of the lobbying of the National Rifle Association (NRA). Although more states have passed so-called red flag laws since the Parkland shooting,[46] NRA-backed legislation has also advanced in many state legislatures.[47] CDC research on gun violence has been stymied by Congress since 1996[48] and several states have tried to prevent doctors from discussing gun safety with families. A statute in Florida was struck down; less stringent measures in Minnesota, Montana, and Missouri limit data collection but do not prevent physician-patient discussion about gun safety. Since Columbine in 1999, more than 150,000 students have been affected by school shootings, and the impact is just now being studied.[49] This is a controversial and sensitive issue, but media portrayals of guns and gun use on TV, in movies, and in video games inevitably contribute to the problem. Even card-carrying members of the NRA should be able to appreciate that there is no Second Amendment right to viewing media gun violence.

IS MEDIA VIOLENCE MORE HARMFUL THAN MEDIA SEX?

Parents and many professionals are far more concerned about sex than violence in the media, possibly reflecting the historically fraught relationship America has with normal, healthy sexuality and sexual behavior. Lack of comprehensive sex education in schools, refusal to provide birth control or condoms in schools and communities, and the incongruity of pornography available on every platform all define a society confused and fearful of sex. In his majority decision in the California video game case (*Brown v Entertainment Merchants Association*), Justice Scalia said that it is appropriate to regulate the sale of *Playboy* magazine to underage youth but not the sale of extremely violent video games.

I GREW UP WATCHING VIOLENT TELEVISION AND MOVIES; WHY AM I NOT AGGRESSIVE OR VIOLENT?

Adults like to believe that they are immune to effects of media, including effects of media violence, advertising, and more. However, this is a perfect example of the third-person effect: everyone else is susceptible, but not me. Quantifying the impact of years of violent portrayals, on the news, in movies, on TV, cannot be done accurately, but imagine the steady drip, drip, drip of media violence, below a conscious level, but affecting people's empathy and beliefs. As stated previously, real-life aggression and violence is complicated, with many, often-related factors.

ARE CARTOONS HARMFUL?

Especially for young children with a less firm grip on reality versus fantasy, cartoon violence has potential harmful effects, just not as significantly as more realistic portrayals. Children learn from attractive characters, whether animal, person, or animated. Scripts for behavior may be accessible from a cartoon character. Cartoons feature plenty of violent scenes (eg, Road Runner and Wily Coyote, dying a thousand deaths) or poignant scenes (eg, Bambi, whose mother was shot and killed off camera).[27]

IS THERE SUCH A THING AS PROSOCIAL VIOLENCE?

To date, there are no published studies addressing whether or not video game violence can be prosocial (modeling and teaching important life lessons about empathy and tolerance). Although numerous studies have documented that shows such as Mr. Rogers' Neighborhood, Daniel Tiger's Neighborhood, and Sesame Street do encourage children to behave in prosocial ways, it is worthwhile noting that they are all explicitly nonviolent. Some children's TV programs with violent content (superhero shows) offer a prosocial lesson at the end, hoping that this will be the takeaway message for young viewers. A few studies done years ago showed that children were often confused about prosocial messages (or the messages were missed entirely): "In other words, the superhero's violent behavior was more salient than his prosocial words were."[3] This outcome was not surprising: violence perpetrated by a good guy and shown to be justified and socially acceptable may be strongly reinforcing to children.[3]

A 2019 review of video games and apps by the Society for Research on Development found a paucity of behavioral studies on older children and preteens but highlighted the positive impact digital games can have on executive functioning, mental and mathematical skills, attention, and problem-solving. For teens, the limited research shows positive influences on perceptual, motor, and cognitive skills but the society acknowledges the negative impact of violent video games.

WHAT DID THE UNITED STATES SUPREME COURT HAVE TO SAY ABOUT MEDIA VIOLENCE?

In 2011, a California case was heard by the Supreme Court to determine whether the sale of violent video games should be restricted. The court, voting 7 to 2, rejected the state's argument that video game violence presented a risk to children.[8] Invoking First Amendment protection, the Court opined that video game violence is protected speech and that the arguments to the contrary presented by California (research-based harm to children) did not represent convincing evidence. Per Justice Scalia: "Like the protected books, plays and movies that preceded them, video games communicate ideas — and even social messages — through many familiar literary devices (such as characters, dialogue, plot, and music) and through features distinctive to the medium (such as the player's interaction with the virtual world)," and therefore video games merit First Amendment protection. The California law would have established a fine for selling violent video games to youth less than 18 years old. It defined violent games as "killing, maiming, dismembering or sexually assaulting an image of a human being" in a way that was "patently offensive," appealed to minors' "deviant or morbid interests" and lacking "serious literary, artistic, political or scientific value." Justice Scalia compared violent video games with Grimm's fairy tales, *The Odyssey*, and other books on high school reading lists.

WHY IS THERE NOT MORE RESEARCH DEVOTED TO MEDIA EFFECTS?

The last serious US government–supported research on media effects on children and adolescents was published in a 1982 National Institute of Mental Health report. At present, dedicated funding for research in this area is lacking. An existing bill in Congress, although unlikely to pass, would provide more than $40 million over several years.[45]

The 10-year-long, NIH-sponsored Adolescent Brain Cognitive Development Study (ABCD study) of children 9 to 10 years old correlated self-reported screen media activity with brain structure neuroimaging. Specific behavioral outcomes were not studied, but "future investigations will need to examine how various forms of screen media activity influence specific psychopathology and cognitive functions." At present, only Common Sense Media and Pew Research Center are doing much media research, and both are primarily assessing usage data, not long-term effects. Researchers at universities continue to provide essential insights into various aspects of media in the lives of children. However, being funded for major projects is competitive and often difficult to achieve and sustain. Other well-funded entities, including private foundations interested in the health and well-being of the nation's children and communities, should consider funding much-needed media research. Clearly, media are going to become more complicated and ubiquitous, and children's lives more saturated. Good research into long-term effects and mitigating strategies is overdue.

SUMMARY

Children and teens live in a media-saturated world. All types of media and platforms are now available, and video gaming continues to be very popular. Video games sales around the world reached $135 billion in 2018.[32] Video games are entertaining and offer opportunities for learning and skill building. At the same time, decades of research finds an association between violence on TV and in movies and real-life childhood and adolescent aggression, both short and long term. Ninety percent of pediatricians and two-thirds of parents either agree or strongly agree that playing violent video games can increase aggressive behavior among children and teens. As Americans grapple with horrific incidents of violence in society, media violence is one factor that could be easily dealt with.

DISCLOSURE

The authors have nothing to disclose.

REFERENCES

1. Minnow N. First speech as FCC chairman. Washington, DC: National Association of Broadcasters; 1961.
2. Anderson CA, Bushman BJ, Bartholow BD, et al. Screen violence and youth behavior. Pediatrics 2017;140:S142–7.
3. Potter WJ. On media violence. Thousand Oaks (CA): Sage Publications; 1999.
4. Committee on Communications. Media violence. Pediatrics 2009;124(5): 1495–503.
5. Council on Communications and Media. Children, adolescents and the media. Pediatrics 2013;132(5):958–61.
6. Bushman BJ, Huesmann LR. Effects of violent media on aggression. In: Singer DG, Singer JL, editors. Handbook of children and the media. 2nd edition. Thousand Oaks (CA): Sage; 2012. p. 231–48.

7. Huesman LR. The impact of electronic media violence: scientific theory and research. J Adolesc Health 2007;41(6):S6–13.
8. Strasburger VC, Donnerstein E. The new media of violent video games: yet same old media problems? Clin Pediatr 2013. https://doi.org/10.1177/0009922813500340.
9. Anderson CA, Ihori N, Bushman BJ, et al. Violent video game effects on aggression, empathy, and prosocial behavior in eastern and western countries: a meta-analytic review. Psychol Bull 2010;136(2):151–73.
10. Strasburger VC. The death of childhood: reinventing the joy of growing up. Newcastle-Upon-Tyne (UK): Cambridge Scholars Press; 2019.
11. Anderson CA, Suzuki K, Swing EL, et al. Media violence and other aggression risk factors in seven nations. Pers Soc Psychol Bull 2017;43(7):986–98.
12. Anderson CA, Bushman BJ. Media violence and the general aggression model. J Soc Issues 2018;74(2):386–413.
13. Gerbner G, Gross L. The scary world of TV's heavy viewer. Psychol Today 1976;10(4):41–89.
14. Bushman BJ, Coyne SM, Anderson CA, et al. Risk factors for youth violence: youth violence commission, International Society For Research On Aggression (ISRA). Aggress Behav 2018;44:331–6.
15. Huesman LR. Nailing the coffin shut on doubts that violent video games stimulate aggression: comment on Anderson, et al. Psychol Bull 2010;136(2):179–81.
16. Moyer MW. Yes, violent video games trigger aggression, but debate lingers. Sci Am 2018.
17. APA Task Force on Violent Media. 2015 APA resolution on violent video games 2015. Available at: www.apa.org. Accessed March 27, 2019.
18. Prescott AT, Sargent JD, Hull JG. Meta-analysis of the relationship between violent video game play and physical aggression over time. Proc Natl Acad Sci U S A 2018. https://doi.org/10.1073/pnas.1611617114.
19. Huesman LR, Moise-Titus J, Podolski CL, et al. Longitudinal relations between children's exposure to TV violence and their aggressive and violent behavior in young adulthood: 1977–1992. Dev Psychol 2003;39(2):201–21.
20. Huesman LR, Lagerspetz K, Eron LD. Intervening variables in the television violence aggression relation: evidence from two countries. Dev Psychol 1984;20(5):746–75.
21. Bandura A, Ross D, Ross SA. Transmission of aggression through imitation of aggressive models. J Abnorm Soc Psychol 1961;63:575–82.
22. Teng Z, Nie Q, Guo C, et al. A longitudinal study of link between exposure to violent video games and aggression in Chinese adolescents: the mediating role of moral disengagement. Dev Psychol 2019;55(1):184–95.
23. Snider M. Study confirms link between violent video games and physical aggression. USA Today 2018.
24. Perloff RM. The third person effect: a critical review and synthesis. Media Psychol 1999;1(4):353–78.
25. Cantor J. Media violence. J Adolesc Health 2000;27(2):30–4.
26. Gentile DA, Bender PK, Anderson CA. Violent video game effects on salivary cortisol, arousal, and aggressive thoughts in children. Comput Human Behav 2017;70:39–43.
27. Strasburger VC. Twenty questions about media violence and its effect on adolescents. Adolesc Med State Art Rev 2014;25(2):473–88.

28. Anderson CA, Gentile DA, Dill KE. Prosocial, antisocial, and other effects of recreational video games. In: Singer DG, Singer JL, editors. Handbook of children and the media. 2nd edition. Thousand Oaks (CA): Sage; 2012. p. 249–72.

29. Anderson M. A majority of teens have experienced some form of cyberbullying. Pew Research Center; 2018.

30. Takizawa R, Maughan B, Arseneault L. Adult health outcomes of childhood bullying victimization: evidence from a five-decade longitudinal British birth cohort. Am J Psychiatry 2014;171(7):777–84.

31. Canadian Pediatric Society. Impact of media use on children and youth. Paediatr Child Health 2003;8(5):301–6.

32. Warman P. Newzoo cuts global games forecast for 2018 to $134.9 billion; lower mobile growth partially offset by very strong growth in console segment. Newzoo 2018.

33. Gera E. Americans spent more than $43 billion on video games in 2018. Variety 2019.

34. McAnally HM, Robertson LA, Strasburger VC, et al. A review of 46 years of violence in films. JAMA Pediatr 2013;167(2):195–6.

35. Singer MI, Anglin TM, Song LY, et al. Adolescents' exposure to violence and associated symptoms of psychological trauma. JAMA 1995;273:477–82.

36. Singer MI, Miller DB, Guo S, et al. Contributors to violent behavior among elementary and middle school children. Pediatrics 1999;104:878–84.

37. Holmes M. The sleeper effect of intimate partner violence exposure: long-term consequences on young children's aggressive behavior. J Child Psychol Psychiatry 2013;54:986–95.

38. Council on Communications and Media. Media use in school-aged children and adolescents. Pediatrics 2016;138(5):e20162592.

39. Council on Communications and Media. Media and young minds. Pediatrics 2016;138(5):e20162591.

40. Broadband Search. 51 critical cyberbullying statistics in 2019. Available at: https://www.broadbandsearch.net. Accessed April 15, 2019.

41. Cyberbullying Research Center. Available at: https://cyberbullying.org/facts. Accessed April 15, 2019.

42. Skilling C. CU researchers launch "cyberbullying detector" program for social media. 2018. Available at: https://www.denverpost.com/2018/06/22/social-media-cyberbullying-detector-bullyalert-university-colorado/. Accessed April 1, 2019.

43. Querry K. Piedmont schools turning to technology to help deter bullying, inappropriate behavior. 2019. Available at: https://kfor.com/2019/01/11/piedmont-schools-turning-to-technology-to-help-deter-bullying-inappropriate-behavior/. Accessed April 1, 2019.

44. Simonite T. Schools are mining students' social media posts for signs of trouble. Wired 2018.

45. S.3286 - CAMRA Act. 115th Congress (2017-2018). Available at: https://www.congress.gov/bill/115th-congress/senate-bill/3286/text?format=txt. Accessed April 1, 2019.

46. Goodin E. States taking initiative in passing gun laws. March 2. 2018. Available at: https://abcnews.go.com/Politics/wireStory/states-adopting-gun-seizure-laws-parkland-tragedy-60956510. Accessed April 1, 2019.

47. Keefe J. Since Parkland shooting, NRA-backed bills have advanced in large numbers in state legislatures. 2018. Available at: https://www.newsweek.com/parkland-shooting-nra-bills-states-891647. Accessed April 15, 2019.

48. Kaplan S. Congress squashed research into gun violence. Since then, 600,000 people have been shot. NY Times. 2018. Available at: https://www.nytimes.com/2018/03/12/health/gun-violence-research-cdc.html. Accessed April 15, 2019.
49. Rowhani-Rahbar A, Zatzick DF, Rivara FP. Long-lasting consequences of gun violence and mass shootings. JAMA 2019. https://doi.org/10.1001/jama.2019.5063.

The Health Challenges of Emerging Adult Gay Men

Effecting Change in Health Care

Perry N. Halkitis, PhD, MS, MPH[a,b,c,]*, Anthony J. Maiolatesi, BA[a,d,e],
Kristen D. Krause, MPH[a,f]

KEYWORDS

- Health disparities • Gay men • Sexual minority men • Gay men's health
- Health challenges • Healthcare challenges

KEY POINTS

- Emerging adult gay men are disproportionally burdened by myriad health disparities, spanning multiple domains (eg, mental, physical, and sexual health).
- The health profile of emerging adult men is complicated further by barriers to accessing competent health care.
- Health care provider knowledge on the unique health and health care needs of emerging adult gay men is severely lacking.
- The utilization of a holistic health care paradigm, the addition of staff education and training sessions, and the creation of a welcoming clinical atmosphere and environment are necessary first steps in providing competent health care to populations of emerging adult gay men.

INTRODUCTION

In the United States, lesbian, gay, bisexual, transgender, and queer (LGBTQ) individuals experience a preponderance of health disparities.[1] These health challenges are predicated on the chronic marginalization and discrimination,[2,3] some of which are state sanctioned,[4,5] experienced by the population, coupled with a health care

[a] Center for Health, Identity, Behavior & Prevention Studies, Rutgers School of Public Health, One Riverfront Plaza, Newark, NJ 07102, USA; [b] Department of Biostatistics, Rutgers School of Public Health, 683 Hoes Lane West, Piscataway, NJ 08854, USA; [c] Department of Urban-Global Health, Rutgers School of Public Health, 683 Hoes Lane West, Piscataway, NJ 08854, USA; [d] Department of Social and Behavioral Sciences, Yale School of Public Health, 60 College Street, New Haven, CT 06510, USA; [e] Center for Interdisciplinary Research on AIDS, Yale University, 135 College Street, New Haven, CT 06510, USA; [f] Department of Health Behavior, Society, and Policy, Rutgers School of Public Health, 683 Hoes Lane West, Piscataway, NJ 08854, USA
* Corresponding author. Departments of Biostatistics, Epidemiology and Urban-Global Health, School of Public Health, Rutgers University, 683 Hoes Lane West, Piscataway, NJ 08854.
E-mail address: perry.halkitis@rutgers.edu

Pediatr Clin N Am 67 (2020) 293–308
https://doi.org/10.1016/j.pcl.2019.12.003
0031-3955/20/© 2020 Elsevier Inc. All rights reserved.

workforce that is inadequately prepared to effectively address the specific health needs of the population. These challenges continue even though policy makers have drawn attention to these matters in recent years.[6,7] In effect, it is imperative that health care providers are adequately prepared to meet the health needs of this population.[8]

Addressing the health needs of the LGBTQ population necessitates a thorough understanding of matters related to both sexual identity (also known as sexual orientation) and gender identity.[9] Using and understanding the correct language and terminology as it relates to the identities of LGBTQ people is an essential initial step in providing competent and compassionate medical care. In this regard, it is critical that providers distinguish sexual orientation from gender identity, as these terms are often conflated with one another. Gender identity refers to "a person's innate, deeply felt psychological identification as a man, woman, or something else, which may or may not correspond to the person's external body or assigned sex at birth (ie, the sex listed on the birth certificate)."[10] Terms that are commonly associated with minority gender identities include genderqueer, gender nonconforming, and gender bender, all of which can be used to refer to gender variations that are not typically associated with the dichotomous view of male and female. Sexual orientation refers to "a person's enduring physical, romantic, emotional, and/or spiritual attraction to another person."[10] Examples of sexual identity include gay, lesbian, heterosexual, bisexual, pansexual (ie, a person's attraction toward people regardless of their sex or gender identity), and asexual (ie, a lack of sexual attraction to others). Sexual identity encompasses both attraction and behavior, and is not limited solely to the sexual acts in which one engages. In this regard, ancient Athenian men engaged in same-sex behavior with young boys, but did not espouse a gay identity. As noted by classicist Eva Keuls[11] (pp. 1–2), "homosexuality as practiced by the Athenians was not about an identity, community, or movement; rather, it was part of a larger syndrome which included men's ways of relating to boys, wives, courtesans, prostitutes, and other sexual partners, and, in a larger sense, to both the people of Athens and to the other city-states." In a sense, Athenian homosexuality was about a patriarchy rooted in male dominance, misogyny, and power, and nothing akin to the gay rights movement of the twentieth century. In the end, homosexual behavior is only one sliver of gay identity, an identity that intersects with many other identities that gay men possess.[12,13]

Over the past 30 years and directed by the acquired immunodeficiency syndrome (AIDS) epidemic, there has been an evolution of terminology associated with sexual orientation labels. The term men who have sex with men (MSM) was coined in 1994 by the Centers for Disease Control and Prevention and has often been used in the human immunodeficiency virus (HIV) literature.[14] The argument for its initial use was driven by 2 perspectives: (1) epidemiologists sought to avoid complex social and cultural connotations that may hinder an epidemiologic investigation of disease by using identity-free terms, and (2) social construction suggests that sexualities are products of social processes and that a more textured understanding of sexuality does not assume alignments among identity, desire, and behavior.[14] MSM and, more recently, WSW (women who have sex with women) have become dominant terms in health-related programming and research for sexual minorities.[14] However, using these umbrella terms often implies a lack of gay or lesbian identity with an absence of community and networks in which same-gender relationships mean something more than just sexual behavior.[14] Moreover, the use of these behavioral/epidemiologic terms fails to address the complex synergy that exists between identity and social conditions, effectively diminishing the significance that identity plays in affecting health, and ultimately framing sexual and gender minority individuals as vectors of disease.[14–16] Inherently, being gay is different from being bisexual or pansexual, although the sexual behavior may be the same, the feelings and salience can be quite distinct.

In addition, the umbrella term LGBTQ is limited in considerations of health and health care for this population recently estimated to constitute approximately 4.5% of the US population.[17] The population is not monolithic, and there is great diversity in the life experiences of L, G, B, T, and Q people.[18] Indeed, across these populations, there is even greater diversity when these identities are considered in relation to age, race, ethnicity, culture, gender identity, national origin, and social class, among other factors. In this regard, conceptualizations and frameworks that seek to target the entirety of the LGBTQ population often fail to address the specific and nuanced health challenges and health care needs of subpopulations within the LGBTQ population. For example, it would be inadequate and false to state that HIV is a health disparity that disproportionately affects the LGBTQ population; rather, it is a health disparity in the United States that overwhelmingly burdens gay and bisexual men and transgender women,[19] who are part, but not the totality, of the LGBTQ population.

It is with this idea in mind that the authors further contextualize the ideas presented in the pages to follow. Given the particularities of health challenges facing various segments of the LGBTQ population, efforts herein focus on one segment of the population: gay men. In particular, the authors consider the health challenges faced by gay men who are emerging adults, recognizing that it is during this period that a vast majority of gay men emerge into their sexual identities,[13,20] and that this developmental period is often fraught with risk behaviors[21] that might impact the health profile of these men in the immediate and set the foundation for health issues across the life course.[22]

ADOLESCENCE AND EMERGING ADULTHOOD IN GAY MEN

The psychologist Jeffrey Arnett (2000) conceptualized the developmental state of emerging adulthood to differentiate the period between adolescence and adulthood, which, in Western industrialized nations, encompasses approximately ages 18 to 25. More recently, the period has been expanded to age 29 so as to capture demographic and educational shifts and also due to the financial realities of Millennials, including Millennial gay men, brought about by the economic crash of 2008 to 2009.[23,24] The group that has come to be known as the Queer Generation[13] is challenged to achieve the financial stability and economic security of generations that preceded them. The demarcation of these years as a developmentally significant period emerged from such demographic trends as an increase in the median age at marriage, lengthier periods of formal schooling, and later ages for having a first child. Some 30% of those graduating high school do not attend college,[25] compounded by those who do not complete high school, makes this a challenging period of exploration and self-discovery. Black and Latino emerging adults are especially challenged during this developmental period because of sociocultural stereotypes about the competencies of minority youth.[26] There has also been a sharp decline in employment opportunities for those with only a high school education, and recent data note that 65.8% of those ages 20 to 24 do not have a college degree.[27] Although there is no longer a lock-step pattern to this period of development, those who successfully negotiate more of the tasks as they transition from the adolescence period, including their education, will experience greater well-being than those who falter and stall.[28]

For gay men, the period of emerging adulthood is a highly vulnerable period in which the confluence of sexual risk taking, drug use, mental health burden, incarceration, and other risk conditions,[29–31] precipitated by experiences of homophobia and discrimination[32,33] from society at large, as well as racism and hegemonic notions of masculinity within the gay population,[13] compromise health and well-being that may last throughout adulthood.[34,35] All in all, these conditions necessitate that health care providers be adequately prepared to address the health needs of this population; to date, there is evidence that such preparation is lacking,[36] first documented in the seminal work of the National Academies.[37] The lack of health care workforce preparation often leads to conditions in which these young gay men forgo care.[38] Although the provision of care for emerging adult gay men has improved relative to past generations of gay men, who were pathologized due to their sexual identity being categorized as a mental illness, invisible to health care providers because of fear of discrimination, or neglected because they were afflicted with AIDS, the conditions are still far from ideal.[39]

HEALTH CHALLENGES FACED BY YOUNG AND EMERGING ADULT GAY MEN

The emergence of the AIDS epidemic in the later twentieth century engendered an unprecedented public health focus on the health and health care needs of gay men.[40] Accordingly, a wave of biomedical and social science emerged that clearly demonstrated the extent to which gay men, including emerging adult gay men, are disproportionally affected by a host of health-related challenges relative to their heterosexual peers.[37,41]

Health disparities among young and emerging adult gay men are well-documented[37,41]; however, the mechanisms and pathways (eg, biological, psychological, and/or sociologic mediators) linking sexual orientation to differential health outcomes remain poorly understood. These health challenges can be conceptualized within a *minority stress framework*,[42–44] which postulates that sexual minority men evidence higher rates of suboptimal health outcomes, relative to heterosexuals, largely because of stress processes stemming from their minority status (eg, sexual identity) membership and the chronic stigmatization of that identity. That is, in addition to general life stressors, emerging adult gay men experience qualitatively unique social stressors because of their sexuality, which accumulate to negatively impact the health profile of this population. For instance, relative to young heterosexual men, young gay or sexual minority men are significantly more likely to experience childhood victimization (eg, parental psychological and physical abuse),[45,46] school-based/peer victimization,[47] low levels of parental support,[48] and forced homelessness because of their sexuality.[49] As such, the health challenges and inequalities addressed in this article are not causally related to homosexuality or gayness, but, instead, are the reflection of noxious social conditions (eg, social marginalization, exclusion, and structural stigmatization) that work in concert to corrode the health profile of young and emerging adult gay men.[41,50–52]

Mental Health

To date, substantial disparities in mental health have been documented in populations of emerging adult gay men.[43,44,53,54] Indeed, past research suggests that gay men evidence higher rates of psychiatric diagnoses and greater lifetime risk for mood-anxiety-substance use disorders relative to heterosexual men.[55] That is, some studies have shown differential rates or levels of suicidal ideation,[56] suicide attempts,[57–60] social anxiety,[61] self-esteem,[61] body image dissatisfaction,[62–64] alcohol use,[65] eating disorders,[66] cigarette smoking,[67] and illicit substance use[68] as a function of sexual orientation. For instance, in a systematic review of mental health disorders and sexual orientation, King and colleagues[68] documented that, across studies, gay men evidenced greater risk for lifetime prevalence of suicide attempts, lifetime prevalence of depression, and lifetime prevalence of anxiety relative to heterosexuals.

Although many emerging adult gay men may struggle with adverse mental health outcomes and reduced psychological well-being, it is critical to note that certain sub-populations (ie, those who are multiply disadvantaged because of intersecting marginalized identities) may be more at risk than others. For instance, the intersection of racial and sexual identity may predict adverse mental health risk insofar as Choi and colleagues[69] documented an association between discrimination and mental health outcomes such that experiences of racism in the past year were positively associated with adverse mental health outcomes (eg, depression and anxiety) in a population of 1196 African American, Latino, and Asian Pacific Islander MSM. These data highlight the degree to which one marginalized identity (eg, nonheterosexual sexual identity) coupled with a second marginalized identity (eg, nonwhite racial identity) may increase the risk for adverse mental health outcomes.

In addition, Gallo and Matthews' *Reserve Capacity Model* postulates that socioeconomic status (SES) is a worthwhile predictor of health disparities due to the well-documented associations among SES, stress, and health.[70–72] As such, emerging adult gay men from lower SES backgrounds may evidence significantly fewer social and psychological resources with which to manage general and minority stressors, thereby amplifying the risk of adverse mental health outcomes. In support of Gallo and Matthews' model,[72] Storholm and colleagues[73] documented the buffering effect of SES on mental health outcomes in emerging adult sexual minority men, such that sexual minority men of higher SES reported lower scores on depression and posttraumatic stress disorder scales relative to lower SES respondents.

Holistically, these data highlight the degree to which young and emerging adult gay men are susceptible to adverse mental health outcomes; however, clinicians must realize that the susceptibility is not uniform across subpopulations of gay men. Instead, the relation between sexual orientation and adverse mental health susceptibility is significantly moderated by identity intersectionality and the degree of disadvantage stemming from the intersections (for more comprehensive reviews on the application of intersectionality to clinical practice, see van Mens-Verhulst J, Radtke HL, Intersectionality and health care: support for the diversity turn in research and practice, unpublished paper, 2006).[74]

Sexual Health

The most documented and researched health disparity among gay men is HIV. Indeed, gay men make up fewer than 5% of the overall US population,[17] yet account for more than half of those currently living with HIV,[75] and approximately 70% of new HIV infections annually.[76] In addition, sexual minority men are the only population within the United States where rates of new HIV infection remain stable, in lieu of decreasing, each year.[19] For example, in a meta-analysis of US population-based surveys, disease rates of HIV (38–75 times as high) and primary and secondary syphilis (63–109 times as high) were significantly higher for gay men, relative to other men.[74] In addition to HIV and syphilis, gay men are disproportionally burdened by other sexually transmitted infections (STIs),[77] such as bacterial STIs (eg, chlamydia and gonorrhea),[78] human papillomavirus,[79,80] Hepatitis B and C,[81,82] and herpes simplex virus (HSV)-2.[83] STI comorbidity remains a common problem among gay men, with syphilis and HIV coinfection being the most documented comorbidity among this population.[52] Within the population, the preponderance of new infections manifests in black and Latino adolescent and emerging adult gay men (13–24 and 25–34) with a decrease in infection among men in their mid-30s.[84]

Physical Health

A focus on physical health disparities among populations of gay men has lagged behind research in other domains, namely mental and sexual health. Despite this notable lacuna in the literature, recent findings have found sexual orientation to be a robust predictor of adverse physical health outcomes, such as migraine headaches,[85] asthma,[86] cancer-related risk behaviors,[87] and cardiovascular health.[88] Indeed, adolescent gay men are significantly more likely to engage in behaviors that amplify lifetime cancer risk and have long-term physical health consequences relative to heterosexual men, such as smoking, consuming alcohol, using illicit drugs, engaging in risky sexual behaviors, reporting little physical activity, and consuming a diet low in fruits and vegetables.[87] As Rosario and colleagues[87] highlight, many of these health and cancer-related risk behaviors emerge early in the life course of sexual minority men (ie, adolescence), effectively increasing lifetime cancer risk among certain sub-populations of gay men due to earlier engagement in cancer-related risk behaviors.

In addition to behavioral risk factors, gay men have been documented to report lower levels of perceived physical health and higher rates of adverse physical health outcomes. In fact, a Netherlands-based study found that, relative to heterosexual men, gay men reported significantly lower perceptions of general health.[89] Similar findings have been replicated in the United States, with Conron and colleagues[86] documenting that, relative to heterosexuals, sexual minorities were more likely to report asthma, smoking, tension and worry, and activity limitation. More recent work has documented associations between sexual orientation and cardiovascular health such that MSM exhibited elevated cardiovascular risk factors and biomarkers.[88] For instance, MSM exhibited elevations in diastolic blood pressure, C-reactive protein, and pulse rate when compared with heterosexual men. Notably, differences in cardiovascular risk as a function of sexual orientation and gender emerged early, with the mean age of the participants being 28.9 years.[88]

It is important to note that research examining the influence of sexual orientation on physical health is still in its infancy, highlighting that the true magnitude of physical health disparities as a function of sexual orientation remains unknown. However, the preceding data offer preliminary support for the extent to which sexual orientation may be a robust predictor of physical health outcomes and, thus, a clinical focus on gay men's physical health is warranted.

HEALTH CARE CHALLENGES

The myriad health challenges faced by emerging adult gay men are magnified due to hardships in accessing adequate and competent health care that serves the unique needs of this population.[37] Contributing factors to inadequate care include overall lack of provider knowledge on health care needs,[90,91] history of stigmatizing experiences in the health care setting, and discomfort around discussing sexual orientation and/or sexual behaviors.[92–94] Because of these conditions, 18% of LGBTQ Americans avoid receiving health care in fear of being discriminated against or treated poorly by health care providers.[95]

As a result of the discomfort and distrust of health care providers, fragmentation of care is common; research indicates that sexual minority men separate their sexual health care from other forms of health care,[96,97] which can lead to inconsistent and inadequate preventive and/or tertiary care. Integrative models using counseling psychologists have been proposed as a means of ameliorating the effects of this schism in health care access.[98–100] It is for this reason that one goal of the Healthy People 2020 campaign is to "improve the health, safety, and well-being of lesbian, gay, bisexual, and transgender (LGBT) individuals."[101] However, the threatened reversal of protective policies (eg, threats to repeal the Affordable Care Act [ACA] and reinterpret the ACA's antidiscrimination mandate)[102–104] and the removal of sexual and gender identity questions from national health-related surveys by the federal government of the United States since 2016 are clear barriers that undermine the efforts that are sought in the goal of Healthy People 2020.

Negative attitudes toward the LGBTQ population and limited expertise on the particularities of gay men's health create these substandard conditions as emerging adult gay men navigate the health care system. For some, there may be a period of failing to access health care as they emerge into adulthood and migrate from their pediatricians and/or family physicians to providers of their own. Indeed, one study identified that 18.7% of California-based physicians indicated discomfort providing care to gay men,[105] harkening back to the early days of the AIDS epidemic when many gay men were abandoned by their health care providers.[106] These realities emerge in medical school; one study indicated that 15% of medical school students reported mistreatment of LGBT students at their schools, whereas 17% of LGBT medical students reported a hostile learning environment.[107] Implicit preferences for heterosexual people versus lesbian and gay people are pervasive among heterosexual health care providers. Sabin and colleagues[108] report that implicit preferences for heterosexual people versus lesbian and gay people are pervasive among heterosexual health care providers; that implicit preferences for heterosexual women were weaker than implicit preferences for heterosexual men; and that heterosexual nurses held the strongest implicit preference for heterosexual men over gay men. Such implicit bias is also noted in public health and other health professions, as has recently been reported by Halkitis.[109]

Moreover, a number of studies indicate that medical schools are inadequately preparing students to enact effective LGBTQ health care provisions.[110] LGBTQ health care training in undergraduate medical education is limited to approximately 5 hours,[111] ranging from a minimum of 3 to a maximum of 8 hours. Compounding the conditions nested within the health professions are the attitudes of the general public: 30.4% of those polled in one study indicated that they would change providers if they discovered that their provider was gay or lesbian, demonstrating the pervasiveness of LGBTQ stigma in American society.[112]

The aforementioned health care challenges experienced by emerging adult gay men are echoed by the results from a recent mixed-methods study conducted by some of the authors.[90] The study participants, all of whom were emerging adult gay men, sought providers who possessed knowledge of the specific health care needs of gay men, especially with regard to same-sex sexual health, which are deficient in most medical school curricula[113]: "*I definitely could've used a doctor to talk to like a – yeah, a doctor to talk to just about what's healthy, and what's not with gay sex.*" These findings also underscore the extant literature regarding negative provider attitudes: "*The doctor wasn't knowledgeable with the LGBT community… She's never really had gay patients so for her it's kinda new and her reaction was kinda like oh, you're young, right now you shouldn't be having anal sex…It wasn't the reaction I was expecting.*" The social conditions experienced by some of the gay men were indicative of the homophobia of health care providers: "*He's [the doctor] a Muslim… So his thing is he doesn't wanna hear too much about sex with guys on guys. So it really makes it really uncomfortable to talk about it because all I'm gonna get is 'Marry a girl'- …It just comes up all the time because he knows I am gay.*" As a result of such situations, many young gay men turn to sources outside the medical profession for knowledge about their health: "*I've always gotten knowledge of gay men health and about risk and HIV and stuff through outside sources…I feel uncomfortable speaking to my doctor."*

LGBTQ health care centers such as Callen-Lorde in New York City and Fenway Health in Boston provide an important service to emerging adult gay men: *"When I visited the gay center, then they taught me a whole new vocabulary and certain different aspects of myself that I should pay attention to more, which helped me out."* This perspective underscores the need for not only more robust, thorough, and tailored education and training on gay men's health care for medical providers, but it also underscores the need for health care spaces and settings that are affirming of sexual minority individuals.

In addition, economic circumstances might compound the aforementioned matters that undermine the health of gay men. Indeed, LGBT individuals experience higher levels of poverty compared with their heterosexual counterparts.[114,115] Thus, LGBTQ health care access is an economic justice issue.[116] For young emerging adult gay men of the Millennial generation, financial worries reside alongside their concerns about their health and their experiences of loneliness and isolation that function to undermine their health.[117]

ADDRESSING THE HEALTH CHALLENGES OF EMERGING ADULT GAY MEN

Emerging adult gay men are disproportionally burdened by and at an increased risk for health challenges and inequalities spanning multiple health domains (eg, mental, physical, and sexual).[37,41] These health burdens do not occur in isolation; instead, the health profile of emerging adult gay men is defined by a set of co-occurring, co-morbid, and mutually enforcing health problems.[118] As conceptualized by Singer and colleagues[119,120] and adapted for gay men by Stall and colleagues,[118] the *syndemic paradigm* postulates that multiple co-occurring epidemics interact synergistically to modify disease risk, transmission, and progression, and that these syndemic conditions are directed by psychosocial burdens, often emanating from experiences of homophobia and discrimination, experienced by this population. These health disparities are largely directed by social and sexual stigma[6]; when laws and policies, such as marriage equality, are enacted, health conditions, including HIV, are projected to improve for the population of emerging adult gay men.[121]

A holistic health care paradigm has applicability to addressing the health of gay men across the lifecourse.[122,123] In this view, health care services for the LGBTQ population broadly, and for emerging adult gay men specifically, must be (1) holistic in nature addressing the multiplicity of health burdens; (2) understood in relation to the social conditions that exacerbate these health disparities, including the transmission of pathogens (ie, a biopsychosocial perspective); and (3) attend fully to sexual and gender identities in the delivery of care. With regard to the latter, it is imperative that emerging adult gay men do not continue to be invisible to health care providers,[124] as they had been before and for years following the Stonewall Riots, which ignited the LBGTQ civil rights movement.[39] One critical step in ensuring this visibility and chipping away at the otherness young gay men feel is the inclusion of sexual and gender identity on all health care intake forms and electronic records.[125,126] Inclusion of these elements function (1) to communicate openly to the provider the identity of the patient, thus directing the provider to tailor services as needed; (2) to validate the life/lived experiences of the patient; and (3) to diminish the stigma and shame too often felt by LGBTQ people. For emerging adult gay men who are in the process of developing their own sexual identity and enacting strategies to disclose who they are, the addition of these 2 questions on any and all health care forms will function to alleviate the already undue burden of a lifetime of "coming out."[13]

Numerous resources and guidelines[127,128] have emerged in recent time in response to the mounting evidence on the numerous health disparities burdening the lives of emerging adult gay men and the LGBTQ population more broadly, much informed by the approaches postulated by leading medical providers and advocates such as Harvey Makadon and colleagues[129] and organizationally through the National LGBT Health Education Center at the Fenway Institute.[10,129] These efforts advance a set of domains that might impact a positive change in the health care delivery to emerging adult gay men: (1) addressing and developing polices that attend to the well-being of LGBTQ people within health care facilities; (2) creating health care environments that are welcoming; and (3) training staff fully and thoroughly to become more adept at addressing the health of the population. These recommendations are enumerated more fully in the aforementioned guidelines. Briefly, policy strategies include the development or adoption of nondiscrimination polices to protect patients as well as recruiting and/or identifying health care providers and staff with expertise working with sexual minority gay men. Welcoming environments would include the creation of gender-neutral bathrooms and the clear display of relevant LGBTQ literature. Finally, ongoing staff training to address biases (eg, homophobia and heterosexism), intersectionality, and tailored education on gay men's health are essential. All of these elements should be complemented by the development and implementation of intake forms that include the collection of sexual and gender identity information.

SUMMARY

Ultimately, effective health care for emerging adult gay men must be cognizant of the fact that these young gay men are grappling with their sexuality during this period of emerging adulthood, which compounds and exacerbates the multitude of developmental issues that emerge during this stage of life. Second, a holistic approach to the health of emerging gay men must use a biopsychosocial frame[15,130] in understanding health challenges with an eye to how social conditions may shape health and how social and emotional well-being are critically tied to physical well-being. Third, skilled and competent health care providers must further recognize that the population of emerging adult gay men is not monolithic, and that all possess intersectional identities,[3,122,131] necessitating tailored approaches to care that fully consider the role of race, ethnicity, culture, social class, and nation of birth, among other factors. Finally, and importantly, the health of emerging adult gay men is not solely defined by HIV; and although the disease continues to persist in the population, the health of young gay men must be envisioned with a broader and less stigmatizing frame if the nation and those that provide care to gay men are to advance the well-being of current and future populations of gay men.

DISCLOSURE

Research reported in this publication was supported by the National Institute on Drug Abuse of the National Institutes of Health under awards R01DA025537 and 2R01DA025537. The National Institute on Drug Abuse of the National Institutes of Health had no role in development of the study design, collection, analysis, or interpretation of the data, writing of the manuscript, or decision to submit the manuscript for publication. The content is solely the responsibility of the authors and does not necessarily represent the official views of the National Institutes of Health.

Additionally, Anthony Maiolatesi's contribution to manuscript preparation was supported in part by The Yale Center for Interdisciplinary Research on AIDS training program, funded by the National Institute of Mental Health under award number T32MH020031-20.

REFERENCES

1. Meyer IH, Northridge ME. The health of sexual minorities: public health perspectives on lesbian, gay, bisexual and transgender populations. New York: Springer; 2007.
2. Bostwick WB, Boyd CJ, Hughes TL, et al. Discrimination and mental health among lesbian, gay, and bisexual adults in the United States. Am J Orthopsychiatry 2014;84(1):35–45.
3. Halkitis PN, Wolitski RJ, Millett GA. A holistic approach to addressing HIV infection disparities in gay, bisexual, and other men who have sex with men. Am Psychol 2013;68(4):261–73.
4. Hatzenbuehler ML. Structural stigma and the health of lesbian, gay, and bisexual populations. Curr Dir Psychol Sci 2014;23(2):127–32.
5. Hatzenbuehler ML. Social factors as determinants of mental health disparities in LGB populations: implications for public policy. Social Issues Policy Rev 2010; 4(1):31–62.
6. Lim FA, Brown DV Jr, Justin Kim SM. Addressing health care disparities in the lesbian, gay, bisexual, and transgender population: a review of best practices. Am J Nurs 2014;114(6):24–34 [quiz: 35, 45].
7. Mulé NJ, Ross LE, Deeprose B, et al. Promoting LGBT health and wellbeing through inclusive policy development. Int J Equity Health 2009;8(1):18.
8. Rossi AL, Lopez EJ. Contextualizing competence: language and LGBT-based competency in health care. J Homosex 2017;64(10):1330–49.
9. Mayer KH, Bradford JB, Makadon HJ, et al. Sexual and gender minority health: what we know and what needs to be done. Am J Public Health 2008;98(6): 989–95.
10. Fenway Health. Glossary of gender and transgender terms. Boston: Fenway Community Health Cent; 2010.
11. Keuls EC. The reign of the phallus: sexual politics in ancient Athens. Los Angeles (CA): Univ of California Press; 1993.
12. Bowleg L. "Once you've blended the cake, you can't take the parts back to the main ingredients": black gay and bisexual men's descriptions and experiences of intersectionality. Sex Roles 2013;68(11–12):754–67.
13. Halkitis PN. Out in time: from Stonewall to queer, how gay men came of age across the generations. New York: Oxford University Press, USA; 2019.
14. Young RM, Meyer IH. The trouble with "MSM" and "WSW": erasure of the sexual-minority person in public health discourse. Am J Public Health 2005;95(7): 1144–9.
15. Halkitis PN. Reframing HIV prevention for gay men in the United States. Am Psychol 2010;65(8):752–63.
16. Khan S, Khan OA. The trouble with MSM. Am J Public Health 2006;96(5):765–6 [author reply: 766].
17. Newport F. In US, estimate of LGBT population rises to 4.5%. In: Gallup: Politics. 2018. Available at: https://news.gallup.com/poll/234863/estimate-lgbt-population-rises.aspx. Accessed June 29, 2019.
18. Stults CB, Kupprat SA, Krause KD, et al. Perceptions of safety among LGBTQ people following the 2016 Pulse nightclub shooting. Psychol Sex Orientat Gend Divers 2017;4(3):251.
19. Centers for Disease Control and Prevention. Diagnoses of HIV infection in the United States and Dependent Areas—2017, vol. 24. Atlanta (GA): HIV Surveillance Report; 2018.

20. Moreira AD, Halkitis PN, Kapadia F. Sexual identity development of a new generation of emerging adult men: the P18 cohort study. Psychol Sex Orientat Gend Divers 2015;2(2):159.

21. Steinberg L. A social neuroscience perspective on adolescent risk-taking. Developmental Rev 2008;28(1):78–106.

22. Sawyer SM, Afifi RA, Bearinger LH, et al. Adolescence: a foundation for future health. Lancet 2012;379(9826):1630–40.

23. Arnett JJ. Emerging adulthood. A theory of development from the late teens through the twenties. Am Psychol 2000;55(5):469–80.

24. Arnett JJ, Žukauskienė R, Sugimura K. The new life stage of emerging adulthood at ages 18–29 years: implications for mental health. Lancet Psychiatry 2014;1(7):569–76.

25. Bureau of Labor Statistics USDofL. College enrollment and work activity of 2013 high school graduates. Washington, DC: Economic News Release; 2014.

26. Eccles JS, Wigfield A, Byrnes J. Cognitive development in adolescence. In: Weiner IB, editor. Handbook of psychology: developmental psychology, Vol. 6. Hoboken (NJ): John Wiley & Sons Inc; 2003. p. 325–50.

27. Kroeger T, Cooke T, Gould E. The class of 2016: the labor market is still far from ideal for young graduates. Report. Washington, DC: Economic Policy Institute; 2016.

28. Schulenberg JE, Bryant AL, O'Malley PM. Taking hold of some kind of life: how developmental tasks relate to trajectories of well-being during the transition to adulthood. Dev Psychopathol 2004;16(4):1119–40.

29. Halkitis PN, Kapadia F, Siconolfi DE, et al. Individual, psychosocial, and social correlates of unprotected anal intercourse in a new generation of young men who have sex with men in New York City. Am J Public Health 2013;103(5):889–95.

30. Halkitis PN, Moeller RW, Siconolfi DE, et al. Measurement model exploring a syndemic in emerging adult gay and bisexual men. AIDS Behav 2013;17(2):662–73.

31. Halkitis PN, Singer SN. Chemsex and mental health as part of syndemic in gay and bisexual men. Int J Drug Policy 2018;55:180–2.

32. Hatzenbuehler ML, Nolen-Hoeksema S, Erickson SJ. Minority stress predictors of HIV risk behavior, substance use, and depressive symptoms: results from a prospective study of bereaved gay men. Health Psychol 2008;27(4):455–62.

33. Mays VM, Cochran SD. Mental health correlates of perceived discrimination among lesbian, gay, and bisexual adults in the United States. Am J Public Health 2001;91(11):1869–76.

34. Halkitis PN, Kupprat SA, Hampton MB, et al. Evidence for a syndemic in aging HIV-positive gay, bisexual, and other MSM: implications for a holistic approach to prevention and healthcare. Ann Anthropol Pract 2012;36(2):365–86.

35. American Psychological Association, APA Working Group on Health Disparities in Boys and Men. Health disparities in racial/ethnic and sexual minority boys and men. Washington, DC: American Psychological Association; 2018.

36. Gayles TA, Garofalo R. Exploring the health issues of LGBT adolescents. In: Schneider JS, Silenzio VMB, Erickson-Schroth L, editors. The GLMA Handbook on LGBT Health. Praeger: Santa Barbara (CA); 2019. p. 133.

37. Graham R, Berkowitz B, Blum R, et al. The health of lesbian, gay, bisexual, and transgender people: building a foundation for better understanding. Washington, DC: Institute of Medicine; 2011.

38. Griffin-Tomas M, Cahill S, Kapadia F, et al. Access to health services among young adult gay men in New York City. Am J Mens Health 2019;13(1). 1557988318818683.
39. Halkitis PN. The stonewall riots, the AIDS epidemic, and the public's health. Am J Public Health 2019;109(6):851–2.
40. Jonsen AR, Stryker JE. The social impact of AIDS in the United States. Washington, DC: National Academy Press; 1993.
41. Wolitski RJ, Stall R, Valdiserri RO. Unequal opportunity: health disparities affecting gay and bisexual men in the United States. New York: Oxford University Press, USA; 2008.
42. Lick DJ, Durso LE, Johnson KL. Minority stress and physical health among sexual minorities. Perspect Psychol Sci 2013;8(5):521–48.
43. Meyer IH. Minority stress and mental health in gay men. J Health Soc Behav 1995;36(1):38–56.
44. Meyer IH. Prejudice, social stress, and mental health in lesbian, gay, and bisexual populations: conceptual issues and research evidence. Psychol Bull 2003;129(5):674.
45. Balsam KF, Rothblum ED, Beauchaine TP. Victimization over the life span: a comparison of lesbian, gay, bisexual, and heterosexual siblings. J Consult Clin Psychol 2005;73(3):477.
46. Cochran BN, Stewart AJ, Ginzler JA, et al. Challenges faced by homeless sexual minorities: comparison of gay, lesbian, bisexual, and transgender homeless adolescents with their heterosexual counterparts. Am J Public Health 2002; 92(5):773–7.
47. Toomey RB, Russell ST. The role of sexual orientation in school-based victimization: a meta-analysis. Youth Soc 2016;48(2):176–201.
48. Needham BL, Austin EL. Sexual orientation, parental support, and health during the transition to young adulthood. J youth adolescence 2010;39(10):1189–98.
49. Kruks G. Gay and lesbian homeless/street youth: special issues and concerns. J Adolesc Health 1991;12(7):515–8.
50. Hatzenbuehler ML, Phelan JC, Link BG. Stigma as a fundamental cause of population health inequalities. Am J Public Health 2013;103(5):813–21.
51. Link BG, Phelan J. Social conditions as fundamental causes of disease. J Health Soc Behav 1995;Spec No:80–94.
52. Wolitski RJ, Fenton KA. Sexual health, HIV, and sexually transmitted infections among gay, bisexual, and other men who have sex with men in the United States. AIDS Behav 2011;15(1):9–17.
53. Mustanski BS, Garofalo R, Emerson EM. Mental health disorders, psychological distress, and suicidality in a diverse sample of lesbian, gay, bisexual, and transgender youths. Am J Public Health 2010;100(12):2426–32.
54. Plöderl M, Tremblay P. Mental health of sexual minorities. A systematic review. Int Rev Psychiatry 2015;27(5):367–85.
55. Cochran SD, Sullivan JG, Mays VM. Prevalence of mental disorders, psychological distress, and mental health services use among lesbian, gay, and bisexual adults in the United States. J Consult Clin Psychol 2003;71(1):53.
56. Cochran SD, Mays VM. Lifetime prevalence of suicide symptoms and affective disorders among men reporting same-sex sexual partners: results from NHANES III. Am J Public Health 2000;90(4):573.
57. Garofalo R, Wolf RC, Wissow LS, et al. Sexual orientation and risk of suicide attempts among a representative sample of youth. Arch Pediatr Adolesc Med 1999;153(5):487–93.

58. Herrell R, Goldberg J, True WR, et al. Sexual orientation and suicidality: a co-twin control study in adult men. Arch Gen Psychiatry 1999;56(10):867–74.
59. Howard J, Nicholas J. Better dead than gay? Depression, suicide ideation and attempt among a sample of gay and straight-identified males aged 18-24. Youth Stud Aust 1998;17(4):28.
60. Paul JP, Catania J, Pollack L, et al. Suicide attempts among gay and bisexual men: lifetime prevalence and antecedents. Am J Public Health 2002;92(8):1338–45.
61. Pachankis JE, Goldfried MR. Social anxiety in young gay men. J Anxiety Disord 2006;20(8):996–1015.
62. Carper TLM, Negy C, Tantleff-Dunn S. Relations among media influence, body image, eating concerns, and sexual orientation in men: a preliminary investigation. Body Image 2010;7(4):301–9.
63. Frederick DA, Essayli JH. Male body image: the roles of sexual orientation and body mass index across five national US Studies. Psychol Men Masculinity 2016;17(4):336.
64. French SA, Story M, Remafedi G, et al. Sexual orientation and prevalence of body dissatisfaction and eating disordered behaviors: a population-based study of adolescents. Int J Eat Disord 1996;19(2):119–26.
65. Corliss HL, Rosario M, Wypij D, et al. Sexual orientation disparities in longitudinal alcohol use patterns among adolescents: findings from the growing up today study. Arch Pediatr Adolesc Med 2008;162(11):1071–8.
66. Austin SB, Ziyadeh NJ, Corliss HL, et al. Sexual orientation disparities in purging and binge eating from early to late adolescence. J Adolesc Health 2009;45(3):238–45.
67. Corliss HL, Wadler BM, Jun H-J, et al. Sexual-orientation disparities in cigarette smoking in a longitudinal cohort study of adolescents. Nicotine Tob Res 2012; 15(1):213–22.
68. King M, Semlyen J, Tai SS, et al. A systematic review of mental disorder, suicide, and deliberate self harm in lesbian, gay and bisexual people. BMC Psychiatry 2008;8(1):70.
69. Choi K-H, Paul J, Ayala G, et al. Experiences of discrimination and their impact on the mental health among African American, Asian and Pacific Islander, and Latino men who have sex with men. Am J Public Health 2013;103(5):868–74.
70. Gallo LC. The reserve capacity model as a framework for understanding psychosocial factors in health disparities. Appl Psychol Health Well-Being 2009; 1(1):62–72.
71. Gallo LC, de los Monteros KE, Shivpuri S. Socioeconomic status and health: what is the role of reserve capacity? Curr Dir Psychol Sci 2009;18(5):269–74.
72. Gallo LC, Matthews KA. Understanding the association between socioeconomic status and physical health: do negative emotions play a role? Psychol Bull 2003; 129(1):10.
73. Storholm ED, Siconolfi DE, Halkitis PN, et al. Sociodemographic factors contribute to mental health disparities and access to services among young men who have sex with men in New York City. J Gay Lesbian Ment Health 2013;17(3):294–313.
74. Purcell DW, Johnson CH, Lansky A, et al. Estimating the population size of men who have sex with men in the United States to obtain HIV and syphilis rates. Open AIDS J 2012;6:98–107.
75. Centers for Disease Control and Prevention. Monitoring selected national HIV prevention and care objectives by using HIV surveillance data—United States and 6 US dependent areas—2010. Atlanta, Georgia: HIV Surveillance Report; 2012.

76. Centers for Disease Control and Prevention. Monitoring selected national HIV prevention and care objectives by using HIV surveillance data—United States and 6 Dependent Areas—2016. HIV Surveill Supplemental Rep 2018;23(4):1–51.

77. Mojola SA, Everett B. STD and HIV risk factors among US young adults: variations by gender, race, ethnicity and sexual orientation. Perspect Sex Reprod Health 2012;44(2):125–33.

78. Benson PA, Hergenroeder AC. Bacterial sexually transmitted infections in gay, lesbian, and bisexual adolescents: medical and public health perspectives. Paper presented at: Seminars in pediatric infectious diseases. 2005.

79. Dunne EF, Nielson CM, Stone KM, et al. Prevalence of HPV infection among men: a systematic review of the literature. J Infect Dis 2006;194(8):1044–57.

80. Halkitis PN, Valera P, LoSchiavo CE, et al. Human papillomavirus vaccination and infection in young sexual minority men: the P18 cohort study. AIDS Patient Care STDs 2019;33(4):149–56.

81. MacKellar DA, Valleroy LA, Secura GM, et al. Two decades after vaccine license: hepatitis B immunization and infection among young men who have sex with men. Am J Public Health 2001;91(6):965.

82. Memon M, Memon M. Hepatitis C: an epidemiological review. J Viral Hepat 2002;9(2):84–100.

83. Xu F, Sternberg MR, Markowitz LE. Men who have sex with men in the United States: demographic and behavioral characteristics and prevalence of HIV and HSV-2 infection: results from National Health and Nutrition Examination Survey 2001–2006. Sex Transm Dis 2010;37(6):399–405.

84. Centers for Disease Control and Prevention. HIV and African American gay and bisexual men. Published 2019. Available at: https://www.cdc.gov/hiv/group/msm/bmsm.html. Accessed October 17, 2019.

85. Strutz KL, Herring AH, Halpern CT. Health disparities among young adult sexual minorities in the US. Am J Prev Med 2015;48(1):76–88.

86. Conron KJ, Mimiaga MJ, Landers SJ. A population-based study of sexual orientation identity and gender differences in adult health. Am J Public Health 2010; 100(10):1953–60.

87. Rosario M, Corliss HL, Everett BG, et al. Sexual orientation disparities in cancer-related risk behaviors of tobacco, alcohol, sexual behaviors, and diet and physical activity: pooled Youth Risk Behavior Surveys. Am J Public Health 2014; 104(2):245–54.

88. Hatzenbuehler ML, McLaughlin KA, Slopen N. Sexual orientation disparities in cardiovascular biomarkers among young adults. Am J Prev Med 2013;44(6):612–21.

89. Sandfort TG, de Graaf R, Bijl RV. Same-sex sexuality and quality of life: findings from the Netherlands Mental Health Survey and Incidence Study. Arch Sex Behav 2003;32(1):15–22.

90. Griffin M, Krause KD, Kapadia F, et al. A qualitative investigation of healthcare engagement among young adult gay men in New York City: a P18 cohort substudy. LGBT Health 2018;5(6):368–74.

91. Rowan D, DeSousa M, Randall EM, et al. "We're just targeted as the flock that has HIV": health care experiences of members of the house/ball culture. Social Work Health Care 2014;53(5):460–77.

92. Brooks H, Llewellyn CD, Nadarzynski T, et al. Sexual orientation disclosure in health care: a systematic review. Br J Gen Pract 2018;68(668):e187–96.

93. Coleman TA, Bauer GR, Pugh D, et al. Sexual orientation disclosure in primary care settings by gay, bisexual, and other men who have sex with men in a Canadian city. LGBT health 2017;4(1):42–54.

94. Petroll AE, Mosack KE. Physician awareness of sexual orientation and preventive health recommendations to men who have sex with men. Sex Transm Dis 2011;38(1):63.

95. National Public Radio, Robert Wood Johnson Foundation, Harvard TH. Discrimination in America: experiences and views of LGBTQ Americans. Chan School of Public Health; 2017. Available at: https://www.npr.org/documents/2017/nov/npr-discrimination-lgbtq-final.pdf.

96. Koester KA, Collins SP, Fuller SM, et al. Sexual healthcare preferences among gay and bisexual men: a qualitative study in San Francisco, California. PLoS One 2013;8(8):e71546.

97. Schneider JA, Walsh T, Cornwell B, et al. HIV health center affiliation networks of black men who have sex with men: disentangling fragmented patterns of HIV prevention service utilization. Sex Transm Dis 2012;39(8):598.

98. Butler M, Kane RL, McAlpine D, et al. Integration of mental health/substance abuse and primary care. Evid Report Technol Assess (Full Rep) 2008;173:1.

99. Dickson GL, Rinaldi AP. Preventing disparities in primary healthcare for LGBT patients. Prev Couns Psychol Theor Res Pract 2012;4:15–20.

100. Tucker CM, Ferdinand LA, Mirsu-Paun A, et al. The roles of counseling psychologists in reducing health disparities. Couns Psychol 2007;35(5):650–78.

101. Lesbian, gay, bisexual, and transgender health. 2019. Available at: HealthyPeople.gov. Accessed August 1, 2019.

102. Barbot O, Durso LE. Promoting a policy and research agenda to protect lesbian, gay, bisexual, and transgender health in the new political era. LGBT Health 2017;4(4):241–3.

103. Cahill SR, Makadon HJ. If they don't count us, we don't count: Trump administration rolls back sexual orientation and gender identity data collection. LGBT Health 2017;4(3):171–3.

104. Gonzales G, McKay T. What an emerging Trump administration means for lesbian, gay, bisexual, and transgender health. Health Equity 2017;1(1):83–6.

105. Smith DM, Mathews WC. Physicians' attitudes toward homosexuality and HIV: survey of a California Medical Society- revisited (PATHH-II). J Homosex 2007; 52(3–4):1–9.

106. Bayer R, Oppenheimer GM. AIDS doctors: voices from the epidemic: an oral history. New York: Oxford University Press; 2002.

107. Hollenbach AD, Eckstrand KL, Dreger AD. Implementing curricular and institutional climate changes to improve health care for individuals who are LGBT, gender nonconforming, or born with DSD: a resource for medical educators. Washington, DC: Association of American Medical Colleges; 2014.

108. Sabin JA, Riskind RG, Nosek BA. Health care providers' implicit and explicit attitudes toward lesbian women and gay men. Am J Public Health 2015;105(9): 1831–41.

109. Halkitis PN. Stonewall riots — 50 years later, has anything changed? Washington, DC: TheHill.com; 2019.

110. Wittenberg A, Gerber J. Recommendations for improving sexual health curricula in medical schools: results from a two-arm study collecting data from patients and medical students. J Sex Med 2009;6(2):362–8.

111. Obedin-Maliver J, Goldsmith ES, Stewart L, et al. Lesbian, gay, bisexual, and transgender-related content in undergraduate medical education. Jama 2011; 306(9):971–7.

112. Lee RS, Melhado TV, Chacko KM, et al. The dilemma of disclosure: patient perspectives on gay and lesbian providers. J Gen Intern Med 2008;23(2):142–7.

113. Coleman E, Elders J, Satcher D, et al. Summit on medical school education in sexual health: report of an expert consultation. J Sex Med 2013;10(4):924–38.
114. Albelda R, Badgett MVL, Schneebaum A, et al. Poverty in the lesbian, gay, and bisexual community. Los Angeles (CA): The Williams Institute; 2009.
115. Badgett MV, Durso LE, Schneebaum A. New patterns of poverty in the lesbian, gay, and bisexual community. Los Angeles (CA): The Williams Institute; 2013.
116. Redman LF. Outing the invisible poor: why economic justice and access to health care is an LGBT issue. Geo J Poverty L Pol'y 2010;17:451.
117. Halkitis PN, Cook SH, Ristuccia A, et al. Psychometric analysis of the Life Worries Scale for a new generation of sexual minority men: The P18 Cohort Study. Health Psychol 2018;37(1):89–101.
118. Stall R, Friedman M, Catania JA. Interacting epidemics and gay men's health: a theory of syndemic production among urban gay men. In: Wolitski RJ, Stall R, Valdiserri RO, editors. Unequal opportunity: health disparities affecting gay and bisexual men in the United States. New York: Oxford University Press; 2008. p. 251–74.
119. Singer M. AIDS and the health crisis of the US urban poor; the perspective of critical medical anthropology. Social Sci Med 1994;39(7):931–48.
120. Singer M, Bulled N, Ostrach B, et al. Syndemics and the biosocial conception of health. Lancet 2017;389(10072):941–50.
121. Halkitis PN. Obama, marriage equality, and the health of gay men. Am J Public Health 2012;102(9):1628–9.
122. Cook SH, Wood EP, Harris J, et al. Theoretical approaches and policy implications. In: Griffith DM, Bruce MA, Thorpe RJ Jr, editors. Men's health equity A Handbook. New York: Routledge; 2019. p. 343–59.
123. Halkitis PN, Kapadia F, Ompad DC, et al. Moving toward a holistic conceptual framework for understanding healthy aging among gay men. J Homosex 2015;62(5):571–87.
124. Makadon HJ. Ending LGBT invisibility in health care: the first step in ensuring equitable care. Cleve Clin J Med 2011;78(4):220–4.
125. Cahill S, Makadon H. Sexual orientation and gender identity data collection in clinical settings and in electronic health records: a key to ending LGBT health disparities. LGBT Health 2014;1(1):34–41.
126. Halkitis PN. Coming out and the otherness of gay men across generations. QED A J GLBTQ Worldmaking 2019;6(2):109–20.
127. Commission J. Advancing effective communication, cultural competence, and patient-and family-centered care: a roadmap for hospitals. Oakbrook Terrace (IL): Joint Commission; 2010.
128. Gay and Lesbian Medical Association. Guidelines for care of lesbian, gay, bisexual, and transgender patients. San Francisco (CA): Gay and Lesbian Medical Association; 2006.
129. Makadon HJ, Potter J, Goldhammer H. The Fenway guide to lesbian, gay, bisexual, and transgender health. Philadelphia: ACP Press; 2008.
130. Thorpe RJ Jr, Halkitis PN. Biopsychosocial determinants of the health of boys and men across the lifespan. Behav Med 2016;42(3):129–31.
131. Carnes N. Gay men and men who have sex with men: intersectionality and syndemics. In: Wright ER, Carnes N, editors. Understanding the HIV/AIDS epidemic in the United States. Cham (Switzerland): Springer International; 2016. p. 43–69.

Supporting Immigrant Children and Youth
What Pediatricians and Other Clinicians Can Do

Randi Mandelbaum, JD, LLM

KEYWORDS

- Unaccompanied minor • Immigrant child • Migrant child • Asylum
- Special immigrant juvenile status (SIJS) • Trauma

KEY POINTS

- Since 2013, the number of unaccompanied minors and families escaping to the United States has increased dramatically.
- Children are fleeing to the United States for multiple and mixed reasons, including but not limited to, community and family violence, extortion, extreme poverty, persecution, the need for protection, and lack of a caregiver.
- Migrant children and families are arriving in communities throughout the United States with medical, mental health, educational, and legal needs that are not easily met without assistance.
- Pediatric providers are uniquely situated to assist migrant children and may in fact be one of the first professionals to interact with the children and families, who may seek out a doctor when a child becomes ill or needs vaccinations to attend school.
- There are many steps that pediatricians and clinicians can take to make their offices welcoming environments, to treat and support migrant children in their communities, and to connect them with necessary resources and critical information.

INTRODUCTION

Since 2013, the number of children arriving at the southern border of the United States has been escalating, primarily with children from the countries of El Salvador, Guatemala, Honduras, and Mexico. Some of these children are alone, having fled dangerous and/or desperate situations in their home countries. Many also may have endured harrowing and life-threatening journeys to the United States. If they are encountered alone by immigration officials, the children will be designated unaccompanied minors, meaning when they arrive in the United States, they are less than the age of 18 and without a parent or guardian.[1] Other children traveling with a parent or guardian may end up being detained or even separated, if apprehended by immigration officials. Still other children and families may enter undetected.

Child Advocacy Clinic, Rutgers Law School, 123 Washington Street, Newark, NJ 07102, USA
E-mail address: randi.mandelbaum@rutgers.edu

Pediatr Clin N Am 67 (2020) 309–324
https://doi.org/10.1016/j.pcl.2019.12.009
0031-3955/20/© 2019 Elsevier Inc. All rights reserved.

pediatric.theclinics.com

Although there is so much to be troubled about concerning the deplorable and dangerous conditions for children detained at the border,[2] what is not always recognized is that many of these children and families ultimately end up living among us, in our communities. For example, unaccompanied minors are frequently released to family members around the country, while their removal (deportation) cases are pending in immigration courts. Similarly, many families with children are released from detention and permitted to live in the community during the pendency of their removal hearings. These children and families, many of whom have experienced multiple forms of trauma, both in their home countries and on the journey to the United States, have extensive needs (for medical, mental health, educational, and legal services) that are not being met. This piece specifically focuses on what pediatricians and other clinicians can do in their communities to help address the needs of these children.[3]

The article begins with a section that documents the growing number of migrant children and families, explaining why so many children and families are escaping to this country, and describing the processes the children and families face once they arrive, as well as the systems with which they must interact. A discussion on the needs of these migrant children follows, including the importance of trauma-informed services, regular medical care, mental health treatment, and legal representation, which would enable many of the children to stabilize their immigration statuses. The article ends with specific recommendations as to what clinicians can do to assist this population of extremely vulnerable children.

THE NUMBERS

One in every 4 children in the United States either was not born in the United States or lives in a family with 1 or more parents who are foreign born.[4] All of these children are typically referred to as "immigrant children"; a subset are those children, mostly from El Salvador, Guatemala, Honduras, and Mexico, who recently have fled to the United States to escape dangerous and deadly community violence and/or extreme poverty. As is indicated in **Table 1**, since 2013, the number of unaccompanied minors and families escaping to the United States has increased dramatically.[5]

Table 1
Entrance of unaccompanied minors into the United States by year

Year	Number of Unaccompanied Minors Entering the United States
Fiscal year (FY) 2013	38,759
FY 2014	68,541
FY 2015	39,970
FY 2016	59,692
FY 2017	41,435
FY 2018	50,036
FY 2019	76,020

Data from U.S. Customs and Border Patrol. United Stated Border Patrol Southwest Family Subject Unaccompanied Alien Children Apprehensions Fiscal Year 2016. https://www.cbp.gov/newsroom/stats/southwest-border-unaccompanied-children/fy-2016, U.S. Customs and Border Patrol. United Stated Border Patrol Southwest Border Apprehensions by Sector FY2018. https://www.cbp.gov/newsroom/stats/usbp-sw-border-apprehensions (Accessed June 24, 2019), and U.S. Customs and Border Patrol. U.S. Border Patrol Southwest Border Apprehensions by Sector Fiscal Year 2020, https://www.cbp.gov/newsroom/stats/sw-border-migration/usbp-sw-border-apprehensions (Accessed December 15, 2019).

An even greater number of children have fled to the United States with 1 or both of their parents. They are termed a family unit or an "adult with child." As is evident from **Table 2**, the number of arriving families also has risen exponentially in the last few years.[6]

The recent increase in children being separated from their parent or parents at our southern border also bears mentioning. On April 6, 2018, the federal government began what it termed a "Zero-Tolerance" policy.[7] Pursuant to this new protocol, the government mandated that all adults who were apprehended at our southern border attempting to cross into the United States be arrested and sent to jail for the crime of illegal entry. However, even many adults who entered through a Port of Entry and requested asylum, a wholly lawful act, were arrested.[8] Because the children could not be jailed with their parents, the children were separated from the parents, designated unaccompanied minors, and sent to shelters run by the Office of Refugee Resettlement (ORR), which is a unit of the US Department of Health and Human Services.[9] In other words, these children were treated as if they were never with their parents, instead of the actual reality of being harshly separated.

After a public outcry and several lawsuits, the Zero Tolerance policy was retracted on June 25, 2018, and on June 26, 2018, the children were court ordered to be reunified with their parents.[10] However, hundreds of children continue to be separated.[11] As of June 30, 2019, the government reported that an additional 911 children had been separated from their parents since June 2018.[12] In addition, on January 17, 2019, an Inspector General's Report, from the US Department of Health and Human Services, concluded that "thousands" of additional children likely had been separated from their parents from July 1, 2017 to June 26, 2018.[13]

PUSH-AND-PULL FACTORS

As is stated above and reflected in **Table 3**, most children and families are coming from Mexico and the Northern Triangle countries of El Salvador, Guatemala, and Honduras.

The overarching question is *why*. To answer this question, it is necessary to explore the conditions in the "home" countries as well as some of the circumstances driving the children and families to leave. Although there may be multiple or mixed reasons,[14] one of the primary explanations given is the increased community and family violence in the Northern Triangle countries.[15] This violence is due in large part to the heightened presence of gangs and drug cartels and also the pervasiveness of gender-based sexual violence.[16] In fact, for each of the past several years, several cities in El Salvador and Honduras have been labeled as the "Murder Capital of the World."[17] Also, a recent study conducted by the United Nations High Commissioner for Refugees of 404 unaccompanied children from El Salvador, Guatemala, Honduras, and Mexico found that 58% would merit protection and likely qualify as refugees because they were found to be "forcibly displaced" and "suffered or faced harms that indicated a potential or

Table 2 Arriving family units by year	
FY 2016	73,888
FY 2017	73,416
FY 2018	105,770
FY 2019	473,682

Data from U.S. Customs and Border Patrol. U.S. Border Patrol Southwest Border Apprehensions by Sector Fiscal Year 2020, https://www.cbp.gov/newsroom/stats/sw-border-migration/usbp-sw-border-apprehensions. (Last visited Dec. 15, 2019).

Table 3 Unaccompanied minors encountered by fiscal year and country of origin									
Country of Origin	FY 2009	FY 2010	FY 2011	FY 2012	FY 2013	FY 2014	FY 2015	FY 2016	FY 2017	FY 2018
El Salvador	1221	1910	1394	3314	5990	16,404	9389	17,512	11,018	4949
Guatemala	1115	1517	1565	3835	8068	17,057	13,589	18,913	18,364	22,327
Honduras	968	1017	974	2997	6747	18,244	5409	10,468	9386	10,913
Mexico	16,114	13,724	11,768	13,974	17,240	15,634	11,012	11,926	11,926	10,136

https://www.acf.hhs.gov/orr/resource/unaccompanied-alien-children-released-to-sponsors-by-county.
From U.S. Customs and Border Protection. US Border Patrol Southwest Border Apprehensions by Sector FY2016 and 2018. Available at: https://www.cbp.gov/newsroom/stats/southwest-border-unaccompanied-children/fy-2016 and https://www.cbp.gov/newsroom/stats/usbp-sw-border-apprehensions.

actual need for international protection."[18] **Table 4** outlines the "push-and-pull" factors frequently cited as to why children are fleeing to the United States.[19] Unfortunately, it also bears mentioning that many youth also experience violence, including sexual assault, extortion, kidnapping, and extreme food, and even water, depravation, on the journey from their home countries to the United States.[20]

Families (adults with children) are fleeing for similar reasons.[21] Many families are frantic to leave gang-infested neighborhoods, where murder and violence are rampant.[22] Women are escaping abusive relationships, attempting to protect themselves and their young children. Still other families are desperate for a life without hunger and depravation, where they can work and provide for their children.

WHAT HAPPENS WHEN THE CHILDREN AND FAMILIES ARRIVE IN THE UNITED STATES?

Before describing what occurs when a child or family arrives at our border, it is necessary to explain the 3 components of the US Department of Homeland Security (DHS).

Table 4 Push and Pull Factors for fleeing to the United States	
Push Factors	**Pull Factors**
• *Pervasive gang and cartel violence* (including recruitment, sexual and gender-based violence, and extortion of children and families) • *Extreme poverty* • *Family violence* (including child abuse and neglect) • *Lack of state protection* (such as a child protection agency) • *Persecution in the home country'* • *Absence of a caregiver*	• Better educational/economic opportunities in the United States • Presence of caregiver in the United States • Relative safety and security in the United States

Data from Justice for Immigrants, U.S. Conference of Catholic Bishops. Root Causes of Migration. Available at: https://justiceforimmigrants.org/what-we-are-working-on/immigration/root-causes-of-migration/ and UN High Commissioner for Refugees (UNHCR), *Children on the Run: Unaccompanied Children Leaving Central America and Mexico and the need for International Protection*, 13 March 2014, available at: https://www.refworld.org/docid/532180c24.html, and Lorenzen, "The Mixed Motives of Unaccompanied Child Migrants from Central America's Northern Triangle."

The officials at our borders, airports, and ports are part of the unit of DHS known as Customs and Border Patrol (CBP). CBP agents are charged with patrolling our borders and determining who can enter and who cannot.[23] Importantly, our border is defined as both the literal border and the area of land within 100 miles of any actual physical boundary.[24] The Immigration and Customs Enforcement (ICE) unit is responsible for the detention and removal of immigrants who are living in the interior of the United States without any lawful immigration status.[25] Finally, the US Citizenship and Immigration Services (USCIS) is the unit of DHS where immigrants can apply for various benefits, such as lawful permanent residence, asylum, Special Immigrant Juvenile visas, T visas, U visas, and Violence Against Women Act (VAWA) relief.[26]

Although many migrant children fleeing to the United States are apprehended when attempting to cross into this country, those who are not may be living in our communities, "under the radar," but with the constant threat that at any moment ICE may detain them or 1 or more members of their family. For those children who were apprehended at the border by CBP officials, the trajectory of what is likely to occur depends on whether the child came to the United States with a parent or alone.

Unaccompanied Minors

For those children (less than the age of 18 years) who arrive alone, CBP officials will place the child into removal (deportation) proceedings. However, pursuant to federal law[27] and a longstanding federal court consent decree,[28] CBP may not detain a child for more than 72 hours, after which the child must be turned over to the US Department of Health and Human Services, in particular, the unit known as the ORR.[29] Children who arrived alone and are designated as unaccompanied minors as well as children who are separated from their parent by US officials, and who are then treated as unaccompanied minors, are included. The 1 exception is children from Mexico, who likely will be immediately returned to Mexico, unless they have been trafficked or can express a fear of return to Mexico.[30]

During these first 72 hours, before being transferred to the custody of ORR, children are typically held in cages or small overcrowded cells,[31] which are often very cold.[32] Recent reports[33] of how children are treated when they are apprehended help shed light on the horrific and dangerous conditions for children detained at our southern border.[34,35] Moreover, the 3-day limit often is not followed, thus leaving children in these appalling conditions for far longer than 3 days.[36]

While in ORR custody, the child will be placed in various ORR facilities. Typical ORR placements are shelters, transitional foster care placements, residential treatment centers, or secure facilities.[37] Even babies and young children are not permitted to be placed into traditional foster homes. Instead, they are placed in what is called transitional foster care, where they are permitted to sleep in a family home, but must report back to the facility for daytime hours, even if the family is willing to care and keep the child in the home.

Recently, the situation has become even more dreadful. Because of the large number of children arriving at the US southern border, ORR has argued that it is in a "crisis" situation, without sufficient shelters and transitional foster care placements for all the children that require them. Under such circumstances, ORR is permitted to place children in what are termed "temporary influx shelters," which are facilities that are not licensed for the care of children and which tend to be huge, congregate care facilities that are more in line with detention centers, and even prisons, than residential child care facilities. In late 2018, 1 influx center, a tent camp in Tornillo, Texas, was shut down because of "serious safety and health vulnerabilities" that were identified by a federal watchdog agency.[38] Not only were there concerns that children were living in tents and were not being provided any real educational programs, but also it was determined that staff members had not undergone background checks and that there was a serious lack of mental health clinicians.[39] On the heels of Tornillo closing in December 2018, a new massive influx shelter opened in Homestead, Florida, which is an unlicensed, for-profit facility that can house up to 2350 children.[40] Similar concerns to those expressed about Tornillo[41] have been alleged against the Homestead facility,[42] including the harsh treatment of children and allegations of sexual abuse inside the center.[43] Moreover, as of June 2019, there were government plans to open 3 new emergency shelters to house approximately 3000 to 4000 unaccompanied children.[44] The shelters are expected to be located on 2 US military bases and at a facility in South Texas.[45]

In sum, despite clear mandates to place children "in the least restrictive environment based upon their best interest"[46] and ORR policies that are supposedly "based on child welfare best practices,"[47] ORR placements are not what are known to be appropriate placements based on sound child welfare policy. Most children in the custody of ORR are housed in huge congregate care facilities,[48] some housing thousands of children, where they (1) do not go to community schools, (2) are not able to visit with family members, (3) do not always receive appropriate medical and mental health care, (4) are limited in the amount of exercise and fresh air they can get, and (5) are not provided with attorneys.[49] In short, these children who fled to the United States to escape violence and danger in their home countries are being further harmed by the US government.

Fortunately, many children in ORR custody are eventually placed with family. Pursuant to federal statutory provisions, if family members are willing and able to care for unaccompanied minors, then the children should be released to family as expeditiously as possible.[50] Specifically, if there is a family sponsor in this country, meaning a parent or other family member (such as grandparents, aunts, uncles, older siblings, or cousins), ORR must attempt to transfer the child to the care of this "sponsor," provided that it is safe to do so, while the child awaits his or her immigration (deportation) hearing. However, this has been taking longer, often many months, and has become more difficult because ORR is now requiring fingerprints and conducting background checks of all sponsors, even those who are parents.[51] In addition, ORR and ICE also are sharing increasing amounts of information, which can be quite concerning to the sponsor, who also may be undocumented.[52]

Families with Children

Children arriving with at least 1 parent or guardian, who are apprehended at the border and not separated, will also be placed into removal proceedings. Most commonly, these families are initially sent to family detention centers. Some are released rather quickly, at times with the parent under electronic monitoring (ankle bracelet). Other families remain indefinitely. Pursuant to a federal court consent decree and a recent court ruling, children are not permitted to be detained for more than 20 days.[53] However, it is not clear if these court mandates are being followed, because many children remain in family detention centers for far longer than 20 days.[54]

NEEDS OF THE CHILDREN

All of the children are arriving in communities throughout the United States with tremendous needs that are not easily met without assistance. Complicating these needs is the fact that, for many of the children and families, English is not their primary language. In fact, some children have limited Spanish language literacy and/or primarily speak indigenous languages.[55] Accordingly, services must be provided by persons who are fluent in the native language of the children and families, a requirement that can be difficult to meet, because of limited bilingual resources.

Medical Care

All healthy children are in need of regular and preventive medical and dental care, and migrant children are no different.[56] In addition, most of the recently arrived children are behind in their immunizations and may need to catch up in order to be able to attend school.[57] Most schools require tuberculosis (TB) screening and a physical examination, along with the recommended battery of immunizations.[58] A more complicated factor is when a child arrives with a preestablished medical condition (asthma, epilepsy, congenital heart disease, and so forth) that requires ongoing care.[59] Meeting their medical needs can be challenging because the children may not qualify for any health insurance.[60] Thus, there is a need for providers who can provide these services for free or at low cost.

Mental Health Treatment

Second, the children have vast mental health needs, with many in desperate need of quality treatment to begin to overcome the extensive and multiple forms of trauma from which they have suffered.[61] Once again, the lack of health insurance, along with the need for bilingual services, further complicates a dire situation and renders the identification of mental health providers extremely challenging.[62]

Assistance Enrolling in School

The children and families also need assistance enrolling the children into school. Although the law is clear that all children have the right to attend school regardless of their immigration status,[63] the reality is that many schools are turning these children away, because of overcrowding and a lack of bilingual services.[64] Without assistance and a firm understanding of the laws and educational policies, families do not know that they can enroll their children in school.

Legal Services

Finally, the children need free or low-cost legal services both to assist in ensuring that the children have a caregiver who has the authority to meet their needs and to assist the children in stabilizing their immigration status.[65] For example, for those children who are not placed with a parent, it may not be clear who can make medical and educational decisions on behalf of the child. The placement of a child by ORR with a family sponsor, such as an aunt or cousin, does not give this relative caregiver any legal rights or authority to consent to medical care or enroll the child into school. It therefore is important for the caregiver to in some way obtain such authority. How this is achieved will depend on state law, but typical processes may include seeking a court order of custody or guardianship or obtaining a form of power of attorney from 1 or both parents.

In addition, if the children were apprehended by CBP officials at the border, they likely were served with documents notifying them that the government is seeking to deport them and that they are expected to appear in immigration court. Many of the children qualify for 1 or more forms of immigration relief, in other words a path to lawful permanent residence status (a "green card"). However, without an attorney to advocate for this relief, it likely will not happen.[66] Thus, the children desperately need attorneys to represent them in immigration court and to assist them with securing immigration relief. Studies show that when children are provided with attorneys, they are more than 5 times more likely to obtain lawful permanent residence status, their "green cards," than without an attorney to assist.[67]

Common forms of relief to which the children may be eligible are special immigrant juvenile status (SIJS) and asylum. SIJS is a humanitarian form of immigration relief available to children who have been found to be unmarried, under the age of 21, abused, neglected, abandoned, or similar by 1 or both parents, and for whom it would not be in the best interest to return to their country of origin.[68] One complicating aspect of SIJS is that it requires that a child be involved with a state family court so that a state court judge can issue an order with the necessary factual findings.[69] Thus, many children are required to appear in 2 courts, family court and immigration court, something that cannot be successfully accomplished without an attorney. A clinician seeking to screen for SIJS eligibility can simply inquire whether a child is residing with 1 or both parents, and if the child is only living with 1 parent, what are the circumstances that led to this situation.

Asylum is a form of protection granted to persons (adults or children) who have a fear of persecution if they are forced to return to their country of origin.[70] Such fear must be based on the person's race, religion, nationality, political opinion, or membership in a particular social group.[71] To determine if a person might be eligible for asylum, one can ask how the person feels about returning to their native country, whether they have a fear of returning, and if so, the basis of the fear.

In addition to SIJS and asylum, a child also might be eligible for a T visa, U visa, or a visa based on domestic violence (VAWA). For a T visa, the child must have been a victim of trafficking and be able to show that he or she would suffer extreme hardship if returned to his or her home country.[72] For a U visa, the child must show that he or she was the victim of a crime, that he or she suffered substantial physical or mental harm as a result of the crime, and that that he or she cooperated with law enforcement in the investigation or prosecution of the crime.[73] Finally, to be eligible for a visa under the VAWA, the child must have been a victim of domestic violence at the hands of his or her parent and this parent must be a lawful permanent resident or US citizen.[74]

HOW PEDIATRICIANS AND OTHER CLINICIANS CAN HELP

Pediatricians are uniquely situated to assist these vulnerable children and may in fact be one of the first professionals to interact with the children and families, who may seek out a doctor when a child becomes ill or needs vaccinations to attend school.[75] Some recommendations for pediatricians and clinicians who wish to enhance their practices to better meet the needs of migrant children are listed in later discussion.[76]

Best Practice

All medical offices serving children should attempt to create a safe and welcoming atmosphere by ensuring that they have linguistically and culturally appropriate capabilities.[77] Various resources, recommended by the American Academy of Pediatrics[78] and the US Department of Health and Human Services,[79] can be found online.

It also is important that all staff in a given medical office be educated on trauma, not only the signs and symptoms but also how best to treat children who have suffered through multiple forms of trauma so that they have the best chance of coping and healing.[80] Embracing organizational principles of trauma-informed care can help provide staff and clinicians guidance on how to approach traumatized patients and families.[81]

Finally, it is critical that parents and children be assured of confidentiality. Families, whereby at least 1 member of the family is undocumented, may be very sensitive to providing detailed personal information, unless they are guaranteed privacy and truly understand that information provided to a medical professional will not be passed on to various governmental entities. Medical professionals should feel secure in promising such confidentiality based on the protections afforded by the HIPPA (Health Insurance Portability and Accountability Act).[82] Moreover, DHS has maintained its policy that recognizes hospitals and medical facilities as "sensitive locations," assuring that they will not be approached by ICE unless exigent circumstances exist.[83] Even then, medical staff at a hospital or doctor's office does not have to cooperate with any government officials unless they are in possession of a judicial warrant, as opposed to a warrant that is issued by ICE itself.[84]

Role of the Pediatrician/Clinician

Although the above recommendations can be viewed as a baseline for helping to develop trust and rapport needed to effectively serve immigrant families, additional supportive measures can be taken to further address the needs of these children and families. Adopting such practices may be particularly helpful in offices located in areas where there is a high volume of migrant children and families, especially families who may be undocumented or who may have recently arrived in this country after fleeing extreme violence or poverty. These additional services could be as simple as assisting families in making connections in the community, referring children or family members to other professionals, or making recommendations about how to keep their children and families safe.

For recently arrived children, there will be an immediate need to have a comprehensive examination and to ensure that the children are up-to-date with their vaccinations or are on a safe and expeditious path to becoming current. Documentation of their immunization history also will be important for school enrollment. Unaccompanied minors who spent time in ORR shelters typically receive some medical care, usually including TB screening, human immunodeficiency virus testing, mental health screening, and sometimes vaccinations. Children who arrive with family members likely will not have seen a medical provider before arriving in their community in the United States. Initial evaluations should focus on identifying preexisting medical conditions, evaluation for illness/trauma, and facilitating school enrollment. The American Academy of Pediatrics has comprehensive guidance for medical screenings and treatment needs and is a good resource for additional, more detailed information.[85]

Mental health screenings and referrals for mental health treatment also may be warranted to address the trauma from which the children may have suffered, because of conditions in the children's home countries, the fact that they may now be separated from 1 or both parents, as well as what they might have endured on the dangerous journey to the United States.[86] The Pediatric ACEs (adverse childhood experiences) and Related Life-events Screener (PEARLS),[87] developed by the Bay Area Research Consortium on Toxic Stress and Health,[88] is a valuable tool to screen for trauma and trauma-related risk symptoms. "The PEARLS screens for a child's exposure to Adverse Childhood Experiences (ACEs) and other potential risk factors for toxic stress (bullying, community violence, food or housing insecurity, etc.) that may increase a child's risk for negative health outcomes."[89]

In addition, it may be beneficial to have additional referral information available, such as legal services providers, free or low cost medical care, and social service organizations, especially those that serve and support immigrant communities. Literature on the local school enrollment process,[90] along with information about the right of all children to attend school, also would be invaluable.[91]

There are also many families with mixed immigration statuses, meaning that 1 or both parents may be undocumented, but the children may be US citizens, have lawful permanent residence status, or be on the path to having some lawful status. These families often worry about what might happen if 1 or both parents are detained or deported. Many jurisdictions permit parents to delegate a trusted relative or friend with the authority to care for one's children should the parent or parents be detained or deported (often called a power of attorney).[92] Having information about this process readily accessible provides invaluable assistance to families who are feeling fearful and vulnerable. It also can be helpful to advise parents or guardians in these circumstances about the importance of making copies of significant documents, such as birth certificates, passports, and medical and educational records, and ensuring that copies of these papers are maintained in a safe place and/or with a trusted friend or relative. This way, if something should happen to their ability to care for the children, the children's necessary documents will be accessible.

Finally, for those pediatricians who wish to make a significant commitment of time and expertise, there are even more intensive and focused efforts that can be explored. First, many undocumented immigrant children lack health insurance and are not eligible for federally funded health insurance through Medicaid if their parents cannot afford private health insurance. Some states do provide health insurance for low-income children regardless of immigration status,[93] and some provide it in specific[94] circumstances,[95] but many do not permit any coverage. Not only can pediatricians help by providing free or low-cost medical treatment but also pediatricians can help to disseminate information as to who may be eligible for publicly funded health insurance, because there is frequent confusion. For example, in some states, children may be eligible for publicly funded health insurance if they have a pending application for SIJS or for asylum (after 180 days).[96] However, often this information is not widely known. Pediatricians also can participate in advocacy efforts seeking to develop state-funded health insurance programs for all low-income children, regardless of a child's immigration status.[97]

Second, depending on one's locale, there may be shelters and facilities nearby that are housing unaccompanied children through contracts with ORR. Pediatricians interested in treating these children can apply to work with these programs as a medical provider.

Pediatricians and other clinicians also can seek to provide one-time medical examinations of migrant children. These assessments can take two different forms. First, many children seeking asylum require forensic medical and mental health examinations to help document and corroborate the harm they suffered. Medical and mental health professionals can volunteer to be trained and then can conduct these forensic evaluations, along with issuing a report of their findings and conclusions. Two organizations that provide such training are Physicians for Human Rights[98] and Health Right International.[99]

In addition, whenever an adult or child is applying for lawful permanent residence status (a "green card"), a medical examination is required by a licensed civil surgeon.[100] Pediatricians, in practice for more than 4 years, can apply to become certified to conduct these examinations.

Finally, there are some model medical-legal partnerships that have been created,[101] specifically focused on the needs of low-income undocumented immigrant children.[102] "Medical-legal partnerships embed lawyers as specialists in health care settings," so that when "problems are detected, clinical staff can refer patients directly for legal services."[103] A leading model of such a partnership, focused on immigrant children, is Terra Firma in New York, which is a nationally recognized medical-legal partnership and is a collaborative project between Catholic Charities of New York, The Children's Health Fund, and The Children's Hospital at Montefiore.[104]

SUMMARY

All children, no matter where they are born, are deserving of safe and secure upbringing, free of community and family violence, where not only their essential needs are met but also they are able to live lives with unconditional love, optimal educational opportunities, and the ability to explore and achieve to their fullest potential. For migrant children, many obstacles stand in the way of them securing even the most basic of necessities, and many live with the constant threat of being returned to countries where their very lives are in danger, or the fear that 1 day they will return home from school and their mother and/or father will be gone. Although pediatric medical professionals cannot respond to all these issues, they are well situated to assist these vulnerable children. Not everyone may wish or be able to launch an advocacy campaign or create a medical-legal partnership. However, there are many smaller steps that pediatricians and clinicians can take to make their offices welcoming environments, to support migrant children in their communities, and to connect them with necessary resources and critical information.

ACKNOWLEDGMENTS

The author thanks Elissa Frank and Alexa Scarpaci for their exceptional research assistance, and Douglas Bishop, MD, and Joanne Gottesman, Clinical Professor of Law, for their thoughtful and invaluable feedback of earlier drafts.

REFERENCES

1. Homeland Security Act of 2002, 6 U.S.C. § 279(g)(2) (2012).
2. Attanasio C, Burke G, Mendoza M. Attorneys: Texas border facility is neglecting migrant kids. El Paso (TX): AP News; 2019. Available at: https://apnews.com/46da2dbe04f54adbb875cfbc06bbc615.
3. Bishop DS, Ramirez R. Caring for unaccompanied minors from Central America. Am Fam Physician 2014;90(9):656–9.
4. American Academy of Pediatrics. Medical screening and treatment recommendations for newly arrived immigrant children, vol. 2. American Academy of Pediatrics, Immigrant Health Toolkit; 2013. p. 13.
5. U.S. Customs and Border Patrol. United States Border Patrol southwest family subject unaccompanied alien children apprehensions fiscal year 2016. Available at: https://www.cbp.gov/newsroom/stats/southwest-border-unaccompanied-children/fy-2016. Accessed December 15, 2019.
6. U.S. Customs and Border Patrol. U.S. Border Patrol southwest border apprehensions by sector fiscal year 2020. Available at: https://www.cbp.gov/newsroom/stats/sw-border-migration/usbp-sw-border-apprehensions. Accessed December 15, 2019.
7. Office of the Attorney General, Memorandum for federal prosecutors along the southwest border, zero-tolerance for offences under 8 U.S.C. § 1325(a). 2018. Available at: https://www.justice.gov/opa/press-release/file/1049751/download.
8. Satija N. The Trump Administration is not keeping its promise to asylum seekers who come to ports of entry. Austin (TX): Texas Tribune; 2018. Available at: https://www.texastribune.org/2018/07/05/migrants-seeking-asylum-legally-ports-entry-turned-away-separated-fami/.

9. Office of Refugee Resettlement. ORR guide: children entering the United States unaccompanied, introduction. 2015. Available at: https://www.acf.hhs.gov/orr/resource/children-entering-the-united-states-unaccompanied.

10. Ms. L. v. U.S. Immigration & customs Enf't ("ICE"), 310 F. Supp. 3d 1133, 1137 (S.D.Cal. 2018).

11. Shepherd K. Up to 5 migrant children are still separated from their family every day, new government data shows. Washington, DC: Am. Immigration Council; 2019. Available at: http://immigrationimpact.com/2019/06/26/migrant-children-still-separated/#.XfhIbNZKjUr.

12. Jordan M. No more family separations, except these 900. New York Times 2019. Available at: https://www.nytimes.com/2019/07/30/us/migrant-family-separations.html.

13. U.S. Department of Health and Human Services, Office of the Inspector General. Separated children placed in Office of Refugee Resettlement care. U.S. Department of Health and Human Services, Office of Inspector General Issue Brief, OEI-BL-18-00511. Washington, DC; 2019.

14. Lorenzen M. The mixed motives of unaccompanied child migrants from Central America's northern triangle, J. on Migration & Hum. Sec. New York: The Center for Migration Studies of New York; 2017. https://doi.org/10.14240/jmhs.v5i4.107. Available at: https://www.researchgate.net/publication/321582470_The_Mixed_Motives_of_Unaccompanied_Child_Migrants_from_Central_America's_Northern_Triangle.

15. Rosenblum MR, Ball I. Trends in unaccompanied child and family migration from Central America. Washington, DC: Migration Policy Institute; 2016.

16. Labrador RC, Renwick D. Central America's violent northern triangle. New York: Council on Foreign Relations; 2018. Available at: https://www.cfr.org/backgrounder/central-americas-violent-northern-triangle.

17. Rosenblum, Ball. Trends in unaccompanied child and family migration from Central America. Migration Policy Institute; 2016. p. 3.

18. UN High Commissioner for Refugees (UNHCR), children on the run: unaccompanied children leaving Central America and Mexico and the need for international protection. 2014. Available at: https://www.refworld.org/docid/532180c24.html.

19. Lorenzen, "The mixed motives of unaccompanied child migrants from Central America's Northern Triangle," at 754.

20. Shetty S. "Most dangerous journey: what Central American migrants face when they try to cross the border." Amnesty International. Available at: https://www.amnestyusa.org/most-dangerous-journey-what-central-american-migrants-face-when-they-try-to-cross-the-border/. Accessed December 15, 2019.

21. Rosenblum, Ball. Trends in unaccompanied child and family migration from Central America. Migration Policy Institute; 2016. p. 3–5.

22. Ibid., 4 in Ref. 21.

23. U.S. Department of Homeland Security. Border patrol overview. 2018. Available at: https://www.cbp.gov/border-security/along-us-borders/overview.

24. The constitution in the 100-mile border zone. Available at: https://www.aclu.org/other/constitution-100-mile-border-zone. Accessed June 28, 2019.

25. U.S. Department of Homeland Security. Removal. 2018. Available at: https://www.ice.gov/ero/removal.

26. U.S. Citizen and Immigration Services. What we do. 2018. Available at: https://www.uscis.gov/about-us/what-we-do.

27. Trafficking Victims Protection Reauthorization Act ("TVPRA"), 8 U.S.C.A. § 1232(b)(3) (2018).

28. "Flores v. Reno." National Center for Youth Law. Available at: https://youthlaw. org/wp-content/uploads/2015/05/Flores_Settlement-Final011797.pdf. Accessed December 15, 2019.
29. 8 U.S.C.A. § 1232(b)(3).
30. 8 U.S.C.A. § 1232(a)(2)(A).
31. O'Leary L. Children were dirty, they were scared, and they were hungry. The Atlantic 2019. Available at: https://www.theatlantic.com/family/archive/2019/06/ child-detention-centers-immigration-attorney-interview/592540/.
32. Chotiner I. Inside a Texas building where the government is holding migrant children. The New Yorker 2019. Available at: https://www.newyorker.com/ news/q-and-a/inside-a-texas-building-where-the-government-is-holding-immi grant-children.
33. Attanasio C, Burke G, Mendoza M. Attorneys: Texas border facility is neglecting migrant kids. El Paso (TX): AP News; 2019. Available at: https://apnews.com/ 46da2dbe04f54adbb875cfbc06bbc615.
34. Cohen E. Pediatricians share migrant children's disturbing drawings of their time in US custody. Atlanta (GA): CNN Health; 2019. Available at: https://www.cnn. com/2019/07/03/health/migrant-drawings-cbp-children/index.html.
35. Linton JM, Griffin M, Shapiro AJ. Detention of immigrant children. Am Acad Pediatr 2017;139(4):1. American Academy of Pediatrics Policy Statement.
36. Alvarez P. House report: at least 18 immigrant children under the age of 2 were separated from parents for 20 days to 6 months. Atlanta (GA): CNN; 2019. Available at: https://www.cnn.com/2019/07/12/politics/house-oversight-committee-family-separations/index.html.
37. Office of Refugee Resettlement. ORR guide: children entering the United States unaccompanied, introduction." Administration for Children and Families, Section 1.1. 2015. Available at: https://www.acf.hhs.gov/orr/resource/children-entering-the-united-states-unaccompanied.
38. Levinson DR. (Inspector General, Department of Health and Human Services) "The Tornillo influx care facility: concerns about staff background checks and number of clinicians on staff." (A-12-19-20000). Washington, DC: Department of Health and Human Services; 2018. p. 1–7.
39. Ibid., 5-6 in Ref. 38.
40. Department of Health and Human Services. Unaccompanied alien children sheltered at Homestead job corps site. Homestead (FL): U.S. Department of Health and Human Services, Administration for Children & Families; 2016. Available at: https://www.hhs.gov/programs/social-services/unaccompanied-alien-children/homestead-job-corps-site-fact-sheet/index.html.
41. Burnett J. "Inside the largest and most controversial shelter for migrant children in the U.S." NPR, (Feb. 13, 2019 10:13 AM). Available at: https://www.npr.org/ 2019/02/13/694138106/inside-the-largest-and-most-controversial-shelter-for-migrant-children-in-the-u-.
42. Kates G, Donaghue E. "'I have spent a lot of time crying': migrant children describe life at Homestead shelter." CBSN. 2019. Available at: https://www. cbsnews.com/news/migrant-children-describe-life-at-homestead-shelter-in-court-filing/.
43. Codd C. "7th child sex abuse allegation at Homestead migrant shelter." CBS Miami. 2019. Available at: https://miami.cbslocal.com/2019/06/20/child-sex-abuse-allegation-homestead-migrant-shelter/.
44. Sacchetti M. HHS to house thousands of unaccompanied minor migrants on military bases and at Texas facility. Washington Post 2019. Available at: https://www.

washingtonpost.com/immigration/hhs-to-house-thousands-of-unaccompanied-minor-migrants-on-military-bases-at-texas-facility/2019/06/07/a6c2c95c-8938-11e9-a491-25df61c78dc4_story.html?utm_term=.f4f6a142a93a.

45. Ibid., in Ref. 44.
46. TVPRA, 8 U.S.C.A. § 1232(c)(2)(B) (2018).
47. Office of Refugee Resettlement, "ORR Guide: children entering the United States unaccompanied, introduction (2015)," at Section 1.1.
48. Gamboa S. Trump administration cutting education, recreation, legal help at migrant children shelters. NBC News; 2019. Available at: https://www.nbcnews.com/news/latino/trump-administration-cutting-education-recreation-legal-help-migrant-children-shelters-n1014316.
49. Jordan M. Migrant children may lose school, sports and legal aid as shelters swell. New York Times 2019. Available at: https://www.nytimes.com/2019/06/05/us/migrant-children-services.html.
50. "Flores v. Reno." National Center for Youth Law, Section IV. Available at: https://youthlaw.org/wp-content/uploads/2015/05/Flores_Settlement-Final011797.pdf. Accessed December 15, 2019.
51. Office of Refugee Resettlement. ORR fact sheet on unaccompanied alien children's services. 2019. Available at: https://www.acf.hhs.gov/orr/resource/orr-fact-sheet-on-unaccompanied-alien-childrens-services.
52. Ibid., in Ref. 51.
53. Flores v. Lynch, 828 F.3d 898 (9th Cir. 2016).rev'd sub nom.Flores v. Session, No. CV 85-4544-DMG (AGRx), 2018 U.S. Dist. LEXIS 115488, at *8 (C.D. Cal. July 9, 2018).
54. Eagly I, Shafer S, Whalley J, et al. Detaining families: a study of asylum adjudication in family detention. Washington, DC: Am. Immigration Council; 2018. Available at: https://www.americanimmigrationcouncil.org/research/detaining-families-a-study-of-asylum-adjudication-in-family-detention.
55. Jawetz T, Shuchart S. Language access has life-or-death consequences for migrants. Washington, DC: Center for American Progress; 2019. Available at: https://www.americanprogress.org/issues/immigration/reports/2019/02/20/466144/language-access-life-death-consequences-migrants/.
56. Bishop DS, Ramirez R. Caring for unaccompanied minors from Central America. Am Fam Physician 2014;90(9):656, 658-9. Dental care is limited in many countries of origin and significant dental and oral health issues are a common concern.
57. Ibid., 658 in Ref. 56.
58. Ibid., 658 in Ref. 56.
59. Ibid., 658 in Ref. 56.
60. Kaiser Family Foundation. Health coverage of immigrants. 2019. Available at: https://www.kff.org/disparities-policy/fact-sheet/health-coverage-of-immigrants.
61. Bishop DS, Ramirez R. Caring for unaccompanied minors from Central America. Am Fam Physician 2014;90(9):658.
62. Ibid., 657 in Ref. 61.
63. Plyler v. Doe, 457 U.S. 202, 230 (1982).
64. Walker T. How undocumented students are turned away from public schools. NEATODAY; 2016. Available at: http://neatoday.org/2016/04/22/undocumented-students-public-schools/.
65. Kelly ML, Ortiz M. Trump administration's suspension of legal aid for migrant children prompts outcry. NPR; 2019. Available at: https://www.npr.org/2019/

06/07/730758892/trump-administrations-suspension-of-legal-aid-for-migrant-children-prompts-outcr.

66. Egkolfopoulou M. The thousands of children who go to immigration court alone. The Atlantic 2018. Available at: https://www.theatlantic.com/politics/archive/2018/08/children-immigration-court/567490/.

67. Ibid., in Ref. 66.

68. 8 U.S.C.A. § 1101(a)(27)(J)(i) (2014).

69. Ibid., in Ref. 68.

70. 8 U.S.C.A. § 1101(a)(42) (2014).

71. Ibid., in Ref. 70.

72. U.S. Citizenship and Immigration Services. Questions and answers: victims of human trafficking, T nonimmigrant status. Available at: https://www.uscis.gov/humanitarian/victims-human-trafficking-other-crimes/victims-human-trafficking-t-nonimmigrant-status/questions-and-answers-victims-human-trafficking-t-non immigrant-status.

73. U.S. Citizenship and Immigration Services. Victims of criminal activity: U nonimmigration status. 2018. Available at: https://www.uscis.gov/humanitarian/victims-human-trafficking-other-crimes/victims-criminal-activity-u-nonimmigrant-status/victims-criminal-activity-u-nonimmigrant-status.

74. Violence Against Women Act, 8 U.S.A.C. § 1154(a)(1)(A)(iii)(I) (2014).

75. Bishop DS, Ramirez R. Caring for unaccompanied minors from Central America. Am Fam Physician 2014;90(9):658.

76. American Academy of Pediatrics. Medical screening and treatment recommendations for newly arrived immigrant children, vol. 2. American Academy of Pediatrics, Immigrant Health Toolkit; 2013.

77. U.S. Department of Health and Human Services, Office of Minority Health. National standards for culturally and linguistically appropriate services in health care 2001.

78. American Academy of Pediatrics. Medical screening and treatment recommendations for newly arrived immigrant children, vol. 2. American Academy of Pediatrics, Immigrant Health Toolkit; 2013. p. 6.

79. U.S. Department of Health and Human Services. Resources. Available at: https://www.thinkculturalhealth.hhs.gov/resources. Accessed December 15, 2019.

80. Tello M. Trauma-informed care: what it is, and why it's important. Boston: Harvard Medical School; 2018. Available at: https://www.health.harvard.edu/blog/trauma-informed-care-what-it-is-and-why-its-important-2018101613562.

81. U.S. Department of Health and Human Services. Trauma. Available at: https://www.integration.samhsa.gov/clinical-practice/trauma-informed. Accessed December 15, 2019.

82. U.S. Department of Health and Human Services. Your rights under HIPAA. Available at: https://www.hhs.gov/hipaa/for-individuals/guidance-materials-for-consumers/index.html. Accessed December 15, 2019.

83. Morton J. U.S. Department of Homeland Security, Enforcement actions at or focused on sensitive locations 2011.

84. Immigrant Legal Research Center. The basics on ICE warrants and ICE detainers. Washington, DC: Immigrant Legal Research Center; 2017.

85. American Academy of Pediatrics. Medical screening and treatment recommendations for newly arrived immigrant children, vol. 2. American Academy of Pediatrics, Immigrant Health Toolkit; 2013. p. 2.

86. Bishop DS, Ramirez R. Caring for unaccompanied minors from Central America. Am Fam Physician 2014;658.

87. For more information on PEARLS. Available at: https://www.dhcs.ca.gov/provgovpart/Documents/PEARLS_FAQ_1.15.19.pdf.

88. California Department of Healthcare Services. The pediatric ACEs and related life-events screener (PEARLS), frequently asked questions (FAQs). Sacramento (CA): California Department of Health Care Services; 2019.

89. Ibid., in Ref. 88.

90. N.J. Department of Education. Immigrant students and school enrollment. 2015. Available at: https://www.nj.gov/education/bilingual/policy/ImmigrantStudentEnrollment.pdf.

91. Children's Law Clinic. Welcoming immigrant children to school: a report of North Carolina school districts. 2017. Available at: https://law.duke.edu/childedlaw/docs/Policy%20Brief%20-%20Enrollment%20of%20Immigrants.pdf.

92. Alger M, Anthony JM, Arriola II, et al. Protecting assets & child custody in the face of deportation: a guide for practitioners assisting immigrant families. Washington, DC: Appleseed Foundation; 2017.

93. Immigrant Legal Research Center. Medical assistance programs for immigrants in various states. Los Angeles (CA): National Immigration Law Center; 2018.

94. Medicaid and CHIP coverage of lawfully residing children and pregnant women. Baltimore (MD): Centers for Medicare & Medicaid Services; 2019. Available at: https://www.medicaid.gov/medicaid/outreach-and-enrollment/lawfully-residing/index.html.

95. Department of Health and Human Services, Center for Medicare and Medicaid Services. Medicaid and CHIP coverage of "lawfully residing" children and pregnant women. 2010. Available at: https://www.medicaid.gov/federal-policy-guidance/downloads/sho10006.pdf.

96. Medicaid. Medicaid and CHIP coverage of lawfully residing children and pregnant women 2019.

97. Chilton LA, Handal GA, Paz-Soldan GJ. Policy statement: providing care for immigrant, migrant, and border children. Itasca (IL): American Academy of Pediatrics; 2013.

98. Physicians for Human Rights. How you can help asylum seekers. Available at: https://phr.org/issues/asylum-and-persecution/join-the-asylum-network/. Accessed December 15, 2019.

99. Health right international. Volunteer. Available at: http://www.healthright.org/volunteer/. Accessed December 15, 2019.

100. U.S. Citizenship and Immigration services. Designated civil surgeons. Available at: https://www.uscis.gov/tools/designated-civil-surgeons. Accessed December 15, 2019.

101. Scott, SM. "Medical-legal partnerships address social issues affecting patient health." AAP News & Journals Gateway. Available at: https://www.aappublications.org/news/2018/02/05/law020518. Accessed December 15, 2019.

102. National Center for Medical-Legal Partnership. The medical-legal partnership toolkit. 2015. Available at: https://medical-legalpartnership.org/wp-content/uploads/2017/11/MLP-Toolkit-Phases-I-and-II.pdf.

103. National Center For Medical Legal Partnership. About medical-legal partnership. Available at: https://medical-legalpartnership.org/faq/. Accessed December 15, 2019.

104. Terra Firma. What we do. Available at: http://www.terrafirma.nyc. Accessed December 15, 2019.

Child Abuse and Neglect
The Role of the Primary Care Pediatrician

Steven Kairys, MD, MPH[a,b,*]

KEYWORDS

- Child abuse • Physical abuse • Child neglect

KEY POINTS

- Child abuse is a common trauma to children of all socioeconomic backgrounds.
- The physical, cognitive, and mental health effects can be overwhelming and last long into adult life.
- Primary care pediatricians as the advocate and care manager for children who are abused can be extremely important to ameliorate the impact of abuse.
- Primary care pediatricians must be able to recognize the early signs and symptoms of abuse.
- Primary care pediatricians must understand the legal and social aspects of abuse and neglect and stay involved to ensure optimal outcomes for these children.

INTRODUCTION

Child abuse and neglect represents an enormous set of issues for the primary care pediatrician. There is ever increasing recognition of the prevalence of trauma in the lives of so many children and the alarming amount of physical and emotional impact of that trauma in childhood and persisting throughout adulthood.[1] The data are clear that children of the upper and middle classes are not protected from abuse and neglect.[2]

Primary care has yet to incorporate trauma prevention guidance, early screening and identification of trauma and abuse, and care management processes to optimize outcomes for children so affected.

This article discusses the current evidence base about the prevalence and impact of abuse and neglect. It explores the role of the primary care pediatrician in prevention, early detection, care management, and advocacy. It provides examples of evidence-based best practices and a road forward, and focuses on physical abuse and neglect.

a Department of Pediatrics, Hackensack Meridian School of Medicine at Seton Hall, Nutley, NJ, USA; b Department of Pediatrics, Jersey Shore University Medical Center, Neptune, NJ, USA
* Department of Pediatrics, Hackensack Meridian School of Medicine at Seton Hall, 340 Kingsland Street, Nutley, NJ 07710.
E-mail address: steven.kairys@hackensackmeridian.org

Pediatr Clin N Am 67 (2020) 325–339
https://doi.org/10.1016/j.pcl.2019.11.001
0031-3955/20/© 2019 Elsevier Inc. All rights reserved.

Medical child abuse and certainly sexual abuse are no less important but are beyond the scope of this article.

DEFINITIONS

Details of child abuse and neglect definitions[3] differ from state to state statutes, although all contain the following components:

- Physical abuse. Harm or threatened harm to the health or welfare of a child through nonaccidental physical injury. In 12 states, there must be actual injury to the child, not only threatened harm.
- Neglect. In the broadest definition, neglect is the failure of a parent or caretaker to provide the resources necessary for the child to grow and thrive. This can include a lack of food, clothing, shelter, medical care, safety, supervision, and schooling. Neglect is often complicated by poverty and by cultural standards. Poverty as the cause of concerns must be separated from an act of omission depriving the child of supervision or safety. Parental alcohol and drug use is the single most common factor in substantiated neglect in the United States.
- Sexual abuse. This refers to the use of inducement or coercion of a child to engage in sexually explicit conduct. This includes incest and rape but also includes pornography, simulated activities of a sexual nature. In most states it also includes human trafficking, prostitution by a child, having a child engaged in sexual activity in filming for commercial purposes.
- Emotional abuse. Although all forms of child abuse have the potential to cause emotional harm, certain acts impact only emotional health. Examples include chronic belittling, terrorizing, mis-socializing, resulting in mood disorders, aggressiveness, posttraumatic stress disorder, and personality disorder.

These definitions are often complex. Many children are abused while alone; often aged 3 years and under and thus preverbal. Much abuse occurs unwitnessed by any other adult or older child. The definitions are also based on the sequelae of the action and not the action itself. For example, a parent can get angry and throw the child against the wall. The action is itself an assault and, by definition, abusive. However, in 1 scenario the child hits the wall with the shoulder and has no injury or bruise-in a second scenario, or the child's head hits the wall and there is subsequent skull fracture and brain injury. The act is the same, the result quite different. Child abuse and neglect is often characterized by such ambiguity.

EPIDEMIOLOGY OF ABUSE AND NEGLECT

There are 2 major data sources about the prevalence of abuse and neglect. The National Child Abuse and Neglect dataset (NCANDS)[4] contains data on all founded referrals to state Child Protective Services (CPS). For the calendar year 2015, there were 683,487 victims for a rate of 9.2/1000 children. The referral rate to CPS was 55.7/1000 children and the rate was 47.1/1000 for children who were investigated because of a referral. Thus, only 17% of investigated referrals resulted in a substantiation for abuse or neglect. Most of the referrals (66%) came from professional sources, especially education. Children from 0 to 1 years had the highest rate at 25/1000 and also the highest mortality. Most of the victims (75%) suffered neglect; 18% suffered physical abuse and 8.6% suffered sexual abuse. Most of the perpetrators were the parents (77.6%)

The National Incidence Study (NIS)[5] is conducted periodically and collects data on children actually harmed by maltreatment and children endangered whether or not there was resultant harm or injury. It uses community sentinels, professionals working with high-risk children and families to get an on-the-ground sampling of abuse and neglect. The last NIS was conducted in 2010. NIS reported that only 32% of children who were harmed were investigated by CPS.

Even as the NIS serves to expand the numbers, so also are several academic surveys. The University of New Hampshire uses a National Survey of Children Exposed to Violence (NSCEV) process based on actual telephone interviews with caregivers of children 0 to 9 years. The second such survey was published in 2016 and demonstrated a 4.0% risk for physical abuse, 5.6% for emotional abuse, and overall that 12.1% of the sample experienced at least one form of maltreatment. These rates are much higher than even the NIS survey rates.

Finally, Felitti and Anda,[6] using the adverse childhood experiences (ACEs) screening tool for adults being seen at medical clinics at Kaiser Permanente, show even higher numbers of adults stating they were abused and/or neglected at some point in their childhood. Their original studies found that 28.3% of this middle-class sample of adult patients at Kaiser self-reported physical abuse as children; and 14.8% self-reported neglect.

By even the most limited data source, NCANDS reported child abuse is epidemic and, if extended to the rates observed from the NSCEV data or the ACE data, the numbers represent numbers so large that any primary care pediatric practice has to have representative numbers as part of their panel of patients being followed.

THE IMPACT AND CONSEQUENCES OF ABUSE AND NEGLECT

The high incidence and prevalence of abuse and neglect is alarming; even more alarming is the enormous toll it takes on so many child victims.

The literature on consequences is voluminous and all congruent. The impact effects physical health, emotional health, and cognitive and social skills.[7–9] The ACE data are the most extensive with regard to physical health effects, with a logarithmic association between the number of ACEs and the risk for heart and liver disease, high blood pressure, recovery from surgery, years of life.[10,11]

Psychological effects include depression and suicidality, anxiety, posttraumatic stress disorder, attention deficit disorder, poor working memory, poor self-control, learning difficulties, and poor self-esteem. Risks for alcohol and substance abuse are similarly increased as the number of traumas increase.[12]

There is robust evidence for the correlation between abuse and neglect and depression, eating disorders, conduct disorder, and drug use. The data are less strong and more inconsistent for physical disease, such as cardiovascular and lung disease.[13]

The original belief was that the risks were increased because of the lower self-esteem and successes as a child, the use of poor coping strategies including poor eating habits, lack of exercise, smoking, and drug use. It is now evident that, in addition to the psychological impacts, there are also actual physiologic impacts. The brain continues to develop through the teen years and until the mid-20s and that trauma and abuse alter the synaptic development and allow for less prefrontal cortex oversight and more impulsive midbrain involvement in decision making and response to distress.[14]

Not every child victim is doomed to a life of failure and emotional distress. Studies have demonstrated that protective factors already in the child's life or promotable can ameliorate some or much of the negative consequences. Skillsets, successes from sports or other activities, positive peers or parents, stable living environment, learning coping strategies and cognitive behavioral adaptive skills, and other such buffers can greatly limit the damages.[15]

THE ROLE OF THE PEDIATRICIAN: PHYSICAL ABUSE

Primary care pediatricians will often see 25 to 30 children each day and many present with bruises to various parts of their bodies. Most of these are certainly accidental but mixed into the cohort are some children whose bruises are inflicted. Despite the data[16] presented here about young children with inflicted injury having prevalence similar to children presenting with otitis media and that socioeconomic status offers little protection, most pediatrician persist in their belief that few children in their practice are at risk or suffer from abuse.[17]

Moreover, despite the continuing education about child abuse, a recent study found that, even for abusive head trauma, the diagnosis was missed in more than 30% of affected children.[18]

Several new approaches supporting pediatricians to be more sensitive to the indicators for potential abuse have developed. The most important of these are the use of sentinel injuries—minor injuries that carry a high risk for abuse and the risk of increased injury in the future—and also Clinical Prediction Rules (CPR) to connect key history and physical findings to improve early detection of physical abuse. See **Box 1**.

Sentinel injuries seek to alert the pediatrician that certain injuries, for example, bruising in a nonambulatory precruising infant are of concern, no matter what part of the body is injured. A recent study demonstrated that, in the premobile infant, less than 1% presented with bruises of any type.[19] Another study [20] documented that in infants with definitive abuse, 27.5% had had a previous bruise, or "sentinel" injury, and that the primary care doctor was aware of such bruising over 40% of the time. Were all infants with bruising further evaluated with more detailed history, skeletal surveys, and potential reports to child protection, many would be spared the damage of further trauma.

CPR extend the alerts of a sentinel injury to include much more information. The first such CPR for physical abuse was proposed by Pierce[21] in 2010 as TEN-4, that any bruise to the torso, ears, or neck in a child less than 4 years was concerning for physical abuse. This was soon expanded to a more inclusive TEN-4FACESp,[22] which added injury to the frenulum, the angle of the jaw, cheek, eyelids, subconjunctival hemorrhage, and patterned type bruises. One multicenter study found that sensitivity to the rule was 96% and specificity was 87%.[23]

A second CPR relates to risk of inflicted brain injury. The PIBIS[24] (Pittsburgh Infant Brain Injury Score) aim is to detect even mild forms of abusive head trauma. It was

---

Box 1
Clinical Prediction Rules for identification of child physical abuse

1. Any bruising to a nonmobile infant

2. TEN-4
   Bruising in a child less than 4 years that is on the torso (chest, abdomen, back, genitals, or buttocks), ears, or neck

3. TEN-4 FACESp (more sensitive and specific than TEN-4)
   In addition to TEN-4, add bruising to the frenulum, the angle of the jaw, the cheek, the eyelids, or subconjunctival hemorrhage

noted by Jenny and colleagues[25] that even at a children's medical center emergency room that many children with mild head trauma were misdiagnosed with gastrointestinal or viral illness and sent home. PIBIS combines infant age with hemoglobin, head circumference, and physical examination, and has shown a 93% sensitivity.

One more tool for the primary care doctor to more regularly detect early signs of physical abuse is the use of the electronic medical records to incorporate triggers of potential concerns.[26] Thirty triggers were embedded based on the Child Protection Team assessment of abuse protocol; for example, order for a skeletal survey, previous documentation of CPS involvement, bruising, domestic violence, and so forth. The trigger system had a sensitivity of 97% and a specificity of 98% and a negative predictive value of 99.9%. Such trigger methodology could be useful for practices able to adapt their emergency medical response EMR to such purpose.

Many paper and pencil screening questionnaires have been proposed for early detection, but the only one that seems to show promise and an actual ability to decrease reports of child abuse is the SEEK questionnaire,[27] which incorporates the screening tool with physician education, availability of a social worker to help the pediatrician with resources and support for families. Developed by Dubowitz, the model has had demonstrated success in both an inner city residency clinic and also in a group of suburban primary care practices in Maryland.

ROLE OF THE PRIMARY CARE PEDIATRICIAN IN DETECTION AND MANAGEMENT OF CHILD NEGLECT

As noted above, most referrals and substantiations for abuse are for neglect. Much of this stems from the epidemic of parental illicit drug use and alcoholism, which results in failure to provide basic needs to the child or a failure to provide adequate supervision and safety.[28] This can also be part of emotional neglect. Medical Neglect is the failure to provide proper medical care for a child in need of such care; and educational neglect due to a child's persistence absence or delays in attending school.[29]

Unlike the mostly overt visible findings in physical abuse, neglect is harm to a child by the omission of care, by failure to provide the care and nurture necessary for a child to grow and be healthy. It is the most common form of child abuse and may result in the most long-term harm. Neglect affects physical health, cognitive development, social development, and emotional health. Dubowitz and Bennett[30] propose a broad definition: child neglect occurs when a child's basic need in not being met resulting in potential or actual harm. Basic needs include food, clothing, shelter health care, safe supervision, nurturance, education.

Most neglect occurs in the shadow of living in poverty; but poverty does not cause neglect. The risk of neglect, however, highly correlates with poverty with much less neglect in families with adequate income. However, parental substance abuse and maternal depression are 2 common factors in neglect and occur in all families regardless of socioeconomic factors.

There are 2 etiologic models for neglect. The parental deficit model[31] proposes that parental substance abuse, mental health issues, cognitive deficits, cause a failure to parent and resultant harm. The ecological-transactional model[32] proposes that it is the interplay of parental attributes and a nonsupportive environment that work in tandem to accelerate the risk for neglect. Thus, the interplay of the stress of poverty, social isolation, parental inability to monitor or to meet their own needs, all interplay in the chronic dysfunction leading to neglect.

Children may typically present to primary care living in a neglectful environment with inadequate health care, with recurring injuries or ingestions, with school truancy, with depression and anxiety related to inadequate emotional care.

Concerns for neglect are not a reason for an automatic referral to child protection. Pediatricians can become concerned when children present with some of the signs listed above. Pediatricians can also use a screening tool to highlight children at potential risk. The SEEK Parent Questionnaire-R (Appendix) is a mixture of assessing family parenting and social difficulties. A primarily social determinant screen, such as WE CARE[33] can also highlight families at high risk because of major issues with housing or food or personal safety or immigration status.

Pediatricians when confronted with a child where the red flags of neglect (**Box 2**) are raised need to take the time, or to have someone in the office take the time, to better understand the social and parental issues confronting the family. The pediatrician needs to consider both the parents' and the child's needs. Concerns need to conveyed honestly and with compassion. The clinician should recognize family strengths also and use those strengths to help outline a course of action. Determine the family's readiness to change and awareness of the issues; allow them to help discover solutions and potential resources. Plans need to be concrete and simple enough to be attainable. At times, a written contract signed by the parents is one way to assure complete understanding of the plan.

If, however, harm is moderate or serious or if voluntary efforts have been fruitless, especially if parental omissions in care and follow-up are reasons for failure to improve, then child protection services are a vital way to make sure the child is safe.

As with all situations where child protection is asked to become involved, it is the pediatrician's responsibility to inform the parents about the referral and the reasons for the referral. The goals of care are to continue to provide support and advocacy for the child and the involvement of child protection is one more layer of that responsibility.

THE PRIMARY CARE PEDIATRICIAN AND THE PREVENTION OF CHILD ABUSE AND NEGLECT

Anticipatory guidance and primary prevention are cornerstones of primary care and the patient centered medical home (**Box 3**). Bright Futures[34] is the American Academy

---

Box 2
Red flags for child neglect

1. Always hungry
2. The child does not develop as expected, including poor weight gain
3. Lack of attention to medical problems
4. Frequent absenteeism or lateness for school
5. Child steals of hoards food
6. Inappropriate dress for the weather
7. Child is apathetic, does not play or notice people
8. Child demanding of affection
9. Parent seems indifferent to child
10. Parent with substance abuse

> **Box 3**
> **Tools for prevention of child abuse**
>
> 1. Connected Kids: Safe Strong Secure—A program by the American Academy of Pediatrics (AAP)
>   a. Includes 21 handouts for parents and children from early childhood to adolescence
> 2. Practicing Safety—A project sponsored by the AAP
>   a. Includes a set of materials including a toolkit, posters, and handouts
>   b. Topics focus on the major risk factors for child abuse
>   i. Infant crying
>   ii. Maternal depression
>   iii. Parental substance abuse
>   iv. Domestic violence
>   v. Infant and toddler sleep and eating behavior
>   vi. Discipline
>   vii. Toilet training
> 3. A Toolkit for Primary Care Providers—Created by the All Alaska Pediatric Partnership using the Strengthening Families Program framework
>   a. A set of materials and information including self-assessments, resilience and positive discipline brochures and more.

of Pediatrics standard of care manual on educating primary care pediatricians about the specifics of providing those components of care.

Thus, pediatricians have the potential to provide such guidance and support to families in their care that would focus on many of the triggers that escalate the risk for abuse and neglect. Surveys from the AAP have thus far shown that most pediatricians do not regularly provide such guidance.[35]

Practicing Safety,[36,37] a prevention program of the AAP, provides tools and materials to promote such prevention in primary care. The modules target coping with crying, parenting, safety in the care of others, family environment, effective discipline, sleeping and eating and toilet training.

Infant crying is the major trigger for abusive head trauma. Anticipatory guidance, guidance to parents about the colic period and concrete ways to safely respond to excessive crying either in the hospital nursery or the pediatrician's office has clear evidence of effectiveness.[38]

Guidance to families about promoting bonding and attachment and the negative consequences of maternal depression at the early well child visits helps provide a framework for a functional environment around the infant. Likewise, planned discussion about safe and healthy child care and a social network to support families when crises arise diminish the potential for risk of harm from unplanned seeking of infant care.

Anticipatory guidance focused on a safe and nurturing family environment, about the stresses of single parenting and also asking if the parent herself feels safe in the home can introduce the risks to the infant and child of home environments that could become toxic for the child. Witnessed violence has been shown to be at least as damaging to the child as actual abuse to the child.[39]

Few pediatricians have developed an anticipatory approach to discipline that provides a philosophy and a set of tools for positive parenting (**Fig. 1**). Many will discuss time out but not a larger goal of using discipline as an opportunity for social learning. Eighty percent of families[40] still consider physical discipline to be effective despite an ever increasing literature on the negative consequences and the lack of effectiveness. In the experience of this author, a large number of physical abuse occurs because

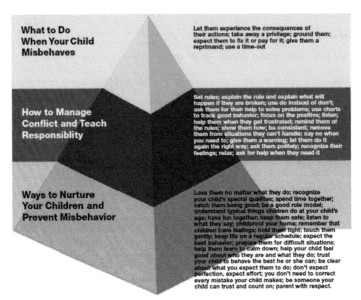

What to Do When Your Child Misbehaves

Let them experience the consequences of their actions; take away a privilege; ground them; expect them to fix it or pay for it; give them a reprimand; use a time-out

How to Manage Conflict and Teach Responsiblity

Set rules; explain the rule and explain what will happen if they are broken; use do instead of don't; ask them for their help to solve problems; use charts to track good behavior; focus on the positive; listen; help them when they get frustrated; remind them of the rules; show them how; be consistent; remove them from situations they can't handle; say no when you need to; give them a warning; let them do it again the right way; ask them politely; recognize their feelings; relax; ask for help when they need it

Ways to Nurture Your Children and Prevent Misbehavior

Love them no matter what they do; recognize your child's special qualities; spend time together; catch them being good; be a good role model; understand typical things children do at your child's age; have fun together; keep them safe; listen to what they say; childproof your home; remember that children have feelings; hold them tight; touch them gently; keep life on a regular schedule; expect the best behavior; prepare them for difficult situations; help them learn to calm down; help your child feel good about who they are and what they do; trust your child to behave the best he or she can; be clear about what you expect them to do; don't expect perfection, expect effort; you don't need to correct every mistake your child makes; be someone your child can trust and count on; parent with respect

Fig. 1. The parenting pyramid. (*Courtesy of* University of Minnesota Extension Service, Minneapolis, MN.)

physical discipline is done as an angry response and the force escalates leaving bruises. The concepts of positive parenting, promoting at the well child visits can promote a discussion and insights to the parents.

Other triggers for abuse include infants not sleeping well, infants and toddlers not eating or being stubborn at meal times and toddlers irregularly toilet training or not training at all. All of these can set up parents to see the toddler as being willful and developmentally capable of volitionally not responding to parental demands. Again, anticipatory guidance and materials about these regularly occurring triggers can promote much more positive and supportive child rearing responses.

THE PRIMARY CARE PEDIATRICIAN AND THE CHILD PROTECTION SYSTEM

Fortunately, most primary care pediatricians are not themselves asked to testify or to partner with the child protection case workers, but they do need to understand the processes and know who to call for advice or to discuss a family in their care.

At its core, child abuse and neglect becomes a legal matter, and courts are asked to judge to merits of the child protection concerns and plans for a child and family and to monitor the plans once adopted.[41] This may involve many months before cases are founded or unfounded. During this period, a safety plan is put in place to assure that the child or children remain safe until a final ruling is made. For some families the risk is low and the family can remain intact with regular contact with the case worker. For higher risk the family will need to be supervised by another relative who remains in the home with the family. If such a person is not available then the next level is relative care with the children moving to a new setting and living with a relative until the case is resolved. As a last resort, for children who have no appropriate relative willing to provide that care, the children are removed and placed into a nonrelative foster care home either as 1 unit or separated into different foster homes if 1 site is not capable of handing all of the children.

Foster care is a necessary evil for many children. Goldstein and colleagues[42] have argued that even a few weeks away from their family feels like a lifetime for too many children. The legal system however grinds slowly and cases can remain on the docket for many months. Some families can afford excellent legal guidance; for many they are at the mercy of a busy office of parental representation and a lawyer that may be overwhelmed by a large caseload to provide effective counsel.

During the often long periods in limbo and then the longer periods when founded cases are under legal scrutiny and regular case worker involvement, there is a need for pediatricians to be comprehensive care managers for these children.

Many pediatric offices will invite a representative from their child protection local office to visit the office so that a mechanism for interaction can be established and a personal connection made to the state service.

AAP has published guidelines[43] for ongoing care for a child who has been maltreated. The guidelines promote the importance of such stability and connection to a child and family, already traumatized, and now going through another period of transition and uncertainty. Recommendations are made for 3 visits in the first 3 months of CPS involvement, whether or not in foster care, and then every 6 months thereafter. The history should include the background and the outcome of the investigation and any child evaluations made during that process.

Because many children traumatized by abuse and neglect will demonstrate behavioral, mood, or cognitive concerns, the pediatrician must be able to understand the issues and assure that a plan is in place to ameliorate the effects of trauma. Using evidence-based assessment tools, such as the SWYC[44] for younger children and the Pediatric Symptom Checklist[45] for older children improves the sensitivity of screening for mental health effects. For older children the CRAAFT[46] screen can be helpful in identifying substance abuse behaviors.

Access and attention to school records allows data on cognitive and academic functioning.

There are also physical consequences of abuse and thus tracking of growth and sexual development are components of the management plan.

Finally, the pediatrician can be beneficial to the child if issues are discovered but are not being addressed or if new concerns become evident as a side effect of the legal process. Pediatricians able to advocate for the best interest of the child are a powerful source of support for the child and are seen by the courts as an impartial voice in a sea of partial voices. A letter to the court can be an effective means of supporting a child in need.

The Pediatrician and the Trauma Informed Office

A pediatrician interested in providing more comprehensive and ongoing services to traumatized children and families can perhaps work best by transforming the office into a trauma informed practice.[47] Transformation must be planned and led by a pediatrician with passion and commitment to the care of children with trauma.

First Step: Realization

An essential first step is to realize that trauma and its impact affects large numbers of children and families in the pediatric practice. This realization needs to be practicewide and not only understood by the providers. The realization changes the way the team members of the practice understand the child and family's issues and behaviors as part of the coping strategies developed to survive adversity.

This realization will lead not only to a constructive response and support for the families but also to efforts to prevent retraumatization by the practice. As important is the secondary realization that being involved with families with so much distress can negatively impact the staff and providers themselves.

Much of trauma informed practice demands that the child and family feel empowered, that there is choice and collaboration in the decisions made, and that children and their families are informed and help develop the plans for care management.

Practice-Based Organizational Changes

Creating a safe environment

Victims of trauma do not feel safe. They are hypervigilant and scan every new environment for evidence of potential danger. They are anxious and untrusting. Helping to create an environment that helps children feel physically, socially, and emotionally safe is fundamental to a trauma informed practice.

A safe physical space is well lit and secure, noise levels are monitored, signage is welcoming and positive, written materials and play materials are engaging and interactive and understandable.

A safe emotional space has staff that engage and are welcoming, positively support the children and families, and treat them with respect. Staff must also be able to stay professional, maintain healthy boundaries with the families, learn how to handle conflict that can arise.

A safe emotional space implies trying to keep to the scheduled times and to openly communicate if delays occur. Staff should be trained to understand some of the cultural differences especially in how those different cultures impact perceptions of trauma and safety and privacy.

Training clinical and nonclinical staff

Training is critical in order for clinicians and staff to be able to work as a team in providing trauma informed care. Training is best done as a team, perhaps by including as part of staff meetings. Training should include content and process components. The office team needs to understand the reasons for the transformation to trauma informed, the background information about the prevalence and impact of trauma to families. There needs to be time and space for the staff discuss their reactions and their own emotional responses to the information.

Process education is the learning of different approaches to initiating positive relationships and supporting families in their care, welcoming and listening, understanding early cues of stress or anxiety and defusing such issues early and effectively.

The whole staff has to embrace the changes for the changes to be impactful. Having 1 or 2 providers or staff that continue with approaches that are not constructive and do not feel safe will dramatically lessen the services that are provided.

Preventing traumatic stress to the staff

It is common for providers and staff that regularly care for children and families who are deeply affected by trauma and toxic stress to internalize that distress. This is often insidious and not readily transparent. Such internalization can lead to fatigue and sadness, poor concentration and effectiveness, illness and absenteeism, emotional detachment, poor social interactions, and physical symptoms and illness. Such burnout is a sad response to trying so hard to help others but it is preventable and can be early detected. For many staff, the impact is increased if that staff has had trauma in their own past, or who are currently living through complicated social and personal difficulties.

Many organizations that deal with trauma work with their staff on prevention approaches, such as mindfulness training, yoga, promoting healthy lifestyles and personal exercise and healthy nutrition. Others promote supervision that is, reflective and directly asks about such trauma effects. Prevention and early detection of this secondary traumatic stress can increase staff morale and improve office function.

Each practice will need to develop its own approach based on its own culture and traditions. However, the approach, the recognition of staff burnout as real and likely is the key factor in the initiation of such efforts.

Clinical Practices

Prevention
Including aspects of trauma prevention into the anticipatory guidance content for well infant and child visits as reviewed above helps to educate families about positive parenting practices, approaches that support attachment, bonding, and promote resilience and strengths.

Practices often have posters that promote such themes, pamphlets and brochures about health child development and child rearing, and staff that are aware of community resources and support services for families with high risk of stress and distress.

Practices need to learn about the abundance of quality community resources that are available to the family-from the child protection to early childhood education and day care resources, to family support networks and organizations.

Screening for trauma
Core to the development of trauma informed care is a process for identifying current or previous trauma in the lives of the children and also the parents. As described elsewhere in this series, the screening for ACEs is the most sensitive tool to pick up those parents and children whose lives have been adversely affected by trauma. The most specific rendition screen is Pediatric ACEs and Related Life Events Screener. It is easy to fill out and score and adaptable to every pediatric office.[48]

The screen allows the pediatrician to better understand the trauma background of the families and to ensure that the family's care adheres to the trauma informed principles.

SUMMARY

Child abuse is epidemic in the United States and occurs to children in all socioeconomic classes. The general pediatrician is in an optimal position to provide preventive guidance to families since they see the young child at least 14 times in the first few years. This frequent engagement also provides the platform for early detection and reporting, which can be lifesaving and/or life altering for many children and families. Practice guidelines are available to the clinician and are regularly updated.[49] The clinician role is not only in prevention and early detection, but also in continuing to care manage the child and the family and help advocate and offer guidance throughout the often difficult paths ahead.

DISCLOSURE

The author have nothing to disclose.

REFERENCES

1. Nemeroff CB, Seligman F. The pervasive and persistent neurobiological and clinical aftermath of child abuse and neglect. J Clin Psychiatry 2013;20:999–1001.

2. Halfon N, Larson K, Son J, et al. Income inequality and the differential effect of adverse child experiences in US children. Acad Pediatr 2017;17(7S):S70–6.
3. Definitions of child abuse and neglect: state statutes. Child Welfare Information Gateway. Children's Bureau ACYF; 2016.
4. Child maltreatment. US Department of Health and Human Services. Administration for Children and Families; 2017.
5. National Incidence Study of child abuse and neglect (NIS-4), 2004-2009. Office of Planning, Research and Evaluation. Administration for Children and Families; 2010.
6. Felitti VJ, Anda RF, Nordenberg D, et al. Relationship of child abuse and household dysfunction to many leading causes of death in adults. Am J Prev Med 1998; 14(4):245–58.
7. Tottenham N. The importance of early experiences for neuro-affective development. Curr Top Behav Neurosci 2016;16:109–29.
8. Doyle C, Ciccheti D. From cradle to grave: the effect of adverse caregiving environment on attachment and relationship throughout the lifespan. Clin Psychol 2017;24(2):203–17.
9. Silverman AB, Reinhenz HZ, Giaconia RM. The long term sequelae of child and adolescent abuse: a longitudinal community study. Child Abuse Negl 1996;20: 709–13.
10. Monnat SM, Chandler RF. Long term physical health consequences of adverse childhood experiences. Sociol Q 2015;56:723–52.
11. Goodqwin RD, Stein MD. Association between childhood trauma and physical disorder among adults in the United States. Psychol Med 2004;34:509–20.
12. MacMillan HL, Fleming JE, Streiner DL, et al. Childhood abuse and lifetime psychopathology in a community sample. Am J Psychiatry 2001;158:1878–83.
13. Fuller-Tomson E, Brennenstuhl S, Frank J. The association between childhood physical abuse and heart disease in adulthood: results from a representative community sample. Child Abuse Negl 2010;34:689–98.
14. Bick J, Nelson CA. Early adverse experiences and the developing brain. Neuropsychopharmacology 2016;41:177–96.
15. Walsh MC, Joyce S, Maloney T, et al. Protective factors of children and families at highest risk of adverse childhood experiences: an analysis of children and families in the growing up in New Zealand data who "Beat the Odds". Wellington (New Zealand): Ministry of Social Development; 2019.
16. Straus MA, Hamby JL. Measuring physical and psychologoical maltreatment of children with the conflict tactic scale. In: Kaufman KG, Jasinki JL, editors. Out of darkness: contemporary research perspectives on family violence. Thousand Oaks (CA): Sage Publications; 1997. p. 119–35.
17. Sege R, Flaherty E, et al. To report or not to report: examination of the initial primary care management of serious childhood injuries. Acad Pediatr 2011;11: 460–6.
18. Letson MM, Cooper JN, Deans KJ, et al. Prior opportunities to identify abuse in children with abusive head trauma. Child Abuse Negl 2016;60:36–45.
19. Sugar NF, Taylor JA, Feldman KW. Bruises in infants and toddlers: those who don't cruise rarely bruise. Arch Pediatr Adolesc Med 1999;153:399–403.
20. Sheets LK, Leach MF, Koszewski IJ, et al. Sentinel injuries in infants evaluated for child physical abuse. Pediatrics 2013;131:701–7.
21. Pierce MC, Kaczor K, Lorenz D, et al. Bruising characteristics discriminating physical child abuse from accidental trauma. Pediatrics 2010;125:67–74.

22. Berger RP, Lindberg MD. Early recognition of physical abuse: bridging the gap between knowledge and practice. J Pediatr 2018;204:16–23.

23. Pierce MC, Kaczor K, Lorenz D, et al. Bruising Clinical Decision Rule (BCDR) discriminates physical child abuse from accidental trauma in young children. San Francisco (CA): Pediatric Academic Society Annual Meeting; 2017.

24. Berger RP, Fromkin J, Herman B, et al. Validation of the Pittsburg infant brain injury score for abusive head trauma. Pediatrics 2016;138:e201–10.

25. Jenny C, Hymel KP, Ritzen A, et al. Analysis of missed cases of abusive head trauma. JAMA 1999;281(7):621–6.

26. Berger RP, Saladino RA, Fromkin J, et al. Development of electronic medical record-based child abuse alert system. J Am Med Inform Assoc 2018;25(2):142–9.

27. Dubowtitz H, Lane W, Semiatin MS, et al. The SEEK model in pediatric primary care: can child maltreatment be prevented in a low risk population. Acad Pediatr 2012;12(4):259–68.

28. Smith VC, Wilson CR. Families affected by parental substance use. Pediatrics 2016;138(2):e1–12.

29. Keeshin BR, Dubowtiz H. Child neglect: the role of the pediatrician. Paediatr Child Health 2013;18(8):e39–43.

30. Dubowitz H, Bennett S. Physical abuse and neglect of children. Lancet 2007;369:1891–9.

31. Hildyard K, Wolfe DA. Cognitive processes associated with child neglect. Child Abuse Negl 2002;31(8):895–907.

32. Daniel B, Taylor J, Scott J. Recognizing and helping the neglected child: evidence-based practice for assessment and intervention. London: Jessica Kingsley Publishers; 2011.

33. Garg A, Toy S, Tripodis Y, et al. Addressing social determinants at well child visits: a cluster RCT. Pediatrics 2015;135(2):e296–303.

34. Hagan J, Shaw JS, Duncan P. Bright futures guidelines. 4th edition. Elk Grove Village (IL): American Academy of Pediatrics; 2017.

35. Sege RD, Siegel BS. Effective discipline to raise healthy children. Pediatrics 2018;142(5):e1–12.

36. Abatemarco DJ, Gubernick RS, LaNoue MD, et al. Practicing safety: a quality improvement intervention to test tools to enhance pediatric psychosocial care for children 0-3. Prim Health Care Res Dev 2018;19(4):365–77.

37. Abatemarco DJ, Karis S, Gubernick R, et al. Expanding the pediatrician's black bag: a psychosocial care improvement model. Jt Comm J Qual Patient Saf 2008;34(2):108–15.

38. Stolz HE, Brandon DJ, Wallace HS. Prevention of shaken baby syndrome: evaluation of a multiple setting program. J Fam Issues 2017;38:2346–67.

39. Stiles MM. Witnessing domestic violence: the effect on children. Am Fam Physician 2002;66(11):2052–60.

40. Straus MA. Beating the devil out of them: corporal punishment in American families. San Francisco (CA): Jossey-Bass; 1994.

41. Schene P. Past, present, and future roles of the child protection system. Future Child 1998;8(1):23–38.

42. Goldstein J, Solnit C, Freud A. Beyond the best interest of the child. New York: MacMillan Press; 1973.

43. Flaherty E, Legano L, Idzerda MD. Ongoing pediatric health care for the child who has been maltreated. Pediatrics 2019;143(4):1–16.

44. Perrin EC, Sheldrick RC. Evidence based milestones for surveillance of cognitive, language and motor development. Acad Pediatr 2013;13(6):577–86.

45. Jelinek MS, Murphy JM, Little M, et al. Use of the PSC to screen for psychosocial problems in pediatric primary care. Arch Pediatr Adolesc Med 1999;153(3): 254–60.

46. Knight JR, Sherritt L, Shrier LA, et al. Validity of the CRAFFT substance abuse screening test among adolescent clinic patients. Arch Pediatr Adolesc Med 2001;156(6):607–14.

47. Menschner C, Maul A. Key ingredients for successful trauma informed care implementation. Princeton (NJ): Center for Health Care Strategies, Inc. Robert Wood Johnson Foundation; 2016.

48. Luckett KM, Wang L. Adverse childhood experiences part 11: ACE screening in pediatrics. San Francisco (CA): Center for Youth Wellness Publication; 2019.

49. Christian C, Committee on Child Abuse and Neglect. The evaluation of suspected child physical abuse. Pediatrics 2015;135(3):e1337–54.

APPENDIX: SEEK PARENT QUESTIONNAIRE-R

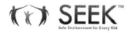 **SEEK**™

Parent Questionnaire - R

Dear Parent or Caregiver: Being a parent is not always easy. We want to help families have a safe environment for kids. So, we're asking everyone these questions about problems that affect many families. If there's a problem, we'll try to help.

Please answer the questions about your child being seen today for a checkup. If there's more than one child, please answer "yes" if it applies to any one of them. This is voluntary. You don't have to answer any question you prefer not to. We will keep this information confidential, unless there's concern that your child is being hurt.

Today's Date: __/__/____   Child's Name: _____

Child's Date of Birth: __/__/____   Relationship to Child: _____

PLEASE CHECK

☐ Yes   ☐ No   Would you like us to give you the phone number for Poison Control?

☐ Yes   ☐ No   Do you need to get a smoke alarm for your home?

☐ Yes   ☐ No   Does anyone smoke at home?

☐ Yes   ☐ No   In the past 12 months, did you worry that your food would run out
                        before you could buy more?

☐ Yes   ☐ No   In the past 12 months, did the food you bought just not last and you didn't have
                        money to get more?

☐ Yes   ☐ No   Do you often feel your child is difficult to take care of?

☐ Yes   ☐ No   Do you sometimes find you need to slap or hit your child?

☐ Yes   ☐ No   Do you wish you had more help with your child?

☐ Yes   ☐ No   Do you often feel under extreme stress?

☐ Yes   ☐ No   Over the past 2 weeks, have you often felt down, depressed, or hopeless?

☐ Yes   ☐ No   Over the past 2 weeks, have you felt little interest or pleasure in doing things?

Thinking about the past 3 months

☐ Yes   ☐ No   Have you and a partner fought a lot?

☐ Yes   ☐ No   Has a partner threatened, shoved, hit or kicked you or hurt you physically in any way?

☐ Yes   ☐ No   Have you had 4 or more drinks in one day?

☐ Yes   ☐ No   Have you used an illegal drug or a prescription medication for nonmedical reasons?

☐ Yes   ☐ No   Other things you'd like help with today: _____

Please give this form to the doctor or nurse you're seeing today. We encourage you to discuss
anything on this list with her or him. Thank you!

©2017, University of Maryland School of Medicine

(*Courtesy of* H. Dubowitz, MD, Baltimore, MD.)

Autism as Representative of Disability

Denise Aloisio, MD[a,b,*], Randye F. Huron, MD[c,d]

KEYWORDS

- Autism • Autism spectrum disorder • Medical home • Vulnerable children
- Care coordination • Early intervention • ABA • Role of physician

KEY POINTS

- Children with autism spectrum disorder (ASD) are vulnerable because of lags in diagnosis, gaps in services, difficulty accessing services, overlooked medical conditions, behavioral difficulties during medical visits, parental stress, bullying, comorbid mental health issues, and variable transitional care moving from adolescence to young adulthood.
- Comprehensive care for children with ASD needs to include earlier recognition of symptoms with timely referral to early intervention services to change the developmental trajectory.
- Creating a medical home in the primary care setting has demonstrated effective care management with emphasis on prevention of secondary comorbidities.
- Primary providers partnering with developmental pediatricians and other specialists can reduce the vulnerabilities of children with ASD by medical advocacy, family education, and appropriate behavior intervention to improve adaptive functioning, self-help skills, and ultimately, independence.

INTRODUCTION

Most recent studies suggest the rate of autism in the United States is 1:59.[1] Primary providers will be caring for more children with autism spectrum disorder (ASD). This population as well as children with other disabilities continues to be vulnerable throughout childhood and adolescence. There can be delays in diagnosis,[2] resulting in lags in therapeutic services. Despite research documenting the benefits of intensive programming,[3] there are large gaps in services owing to lack of funding, available service providers, and misperceptions about effective treatments. School district services vary widely across the country with no clear consensus of best practice for

[a] Hackensack Meridian Health, K. Hovnanian Children's Hospital - Jersey Shore University Medical Center, Division of Developmental Behavioral Pediatrics, Child Evaluation Center, 81 Davis Avenue, Suite 1, Neptune, NJ 07753, USA; [b] Pediatrics, Hackensack Meridian School of Medicine, Nutley, NJ, USA; [c] Hackensack Meridian Health, Joseph M. Sanzari Children's Hospital - Hackensack University Medical Center, Institute for Child Development, 30 Prospect Avenue, Hackensack, NJ 07601, USA; [d] Hackensack Meridian School of Medicine, Nutley, NJ, USA
* Corresponding author. K. Hovnanian Children's Hospital - Jersey Shore University Medical Center, Child Evaluation Center, 81 Davis Avenue, Suite 1, Neptune, NJ 07753.
E-mail address: Denise.Aloisio@Hackensackmeridian.org

Pediatr Clin N Am 67 (2020) 341–355
https://doi.org/10.1016/j.pcl.2019.12.008
0031-3955/20/© 2020 Elsevier Inc. All rights reserved.

preschool and school-aged children. Inadequate educational programs can lead to avoidable learning and adaptive delays, further compounding a child's disability.

Because children with ASD process information differently, they may experience significant sensory difficulties[4] and have excessive reactivity in a medical setting. Medical visits can be compromised, leading to suboptimal care. Medical conditions that lead to increased maladaptive behaviors[5,6] may be overlooked. Recognizing these needs and changing the way providers care for these children can improve outcomes for the child and the family. Parents and caregivers experience high levels of stress in situations in which their child is acting out and when they are not receiving appropriate services to address their needs. Families struggle with the diagnosis, unanswered questions, no real causes, and no specific cures for this lifelong condition.

Stigma still attached to developmental disabilities and special education services affects the way parents may approach the diagnosis and management. Families need to process developmental differences at each new developmental milestone. As the child gets older, differences in functioning skills and the level of supports needed may become more apparent. Comorbid conditions, including attention-deficit/hyperactivity disorder (ADHD), anxiety, depression, and learning disabilities, further contribute to impaired functioning and social isolation.[5] Children with ASD are more susceptible to exclusion by peers, bullying, and abuse.[7–9] Late adolescence and young adulthood bring new challenges with limited educational programming and few opportunities for meaningful vocational experiences.[10] Although the medical and educational systems have made much progress in the care of individuals with ASD, there continues to be a strong need for comprehensive collaborative multidisciplinary care to improve outcomes and provide family supports.

BACKGROUND AND HISTORY

The Story of Intellectual Disability, edited by Michael Wehmeyer,[11] relates the timeline of treatment of those with intellectual disabilities in the 1900s to 2013. In the early 1900s, institutionalization rapidly expanded, reaching capacity in the 1920s. In 1907, Indiana became the first state to pass sterilization laws for those with intellectual disability in state institutions.[11] Physicians encouraged families to place their child in an institution at a young age without waiting to determine the child's developmental potential. Free public education for all children did not become a reality until 1975 with the federal law, Education for All Handicapped Children Act, PL94-142 (now IDEA). The term autism was first introduced in the medical literature in 1943 by Dr Leo Kanner but was not widely understood. In fact, theories of causation suggested the fault lie with the mother.

Despite the original publication in 1952, autism did not appear in the *Diagnostic and Statistical Manual* (*DSM*) until 1980. In 1987, a new addition expanded the criteria, and in 1991, the US Department of Education ruled that a diagnosis of autism qualifies a child for special education services. It was not until 1991 that Asperger syndrome was included in *DSM-IV*, but 22 years later, the definition of autism changed again with *DSM-V*, published in 2013, when the term pervasive developmental disorder and Asperger syndrome were exchanged for ASD, and levels of functioning based on support needed were outlined.[12] Although there was careful consideration of these recommendations by a team of highly qualified specialists with the rationale to clarify the diagnosis, there has also been added confusion, creating a whole population of young adults diagnosed with a condition no longer recognized by the term they have come to understand.

Caring for individuals with ASD requires physicians to be open to the possibilities of tremendous developmental change and be aware of their own bias acquired from previous experiences. A diagnosis of autism 50 or 20 years ago is very different from a diagnosis now. Unlike a bacterial infection or some forms of cancer that are readily identifiable, a diagnosis of autism relies on clinical expertise and medical opinion. What the child looks like at the age of 2 years old in no way predicts where they will be at 21 years of age. It is essential that physicians come to families with an openness to uncertainty, recognizing the dramatic historic changes that have occurred over the past century and conveying hope for optimal developmental progression.

CONSIDERING THE RISING PREVALENCE OF AUTISM

The prevalence rates of autism seem to be rising at an alarming rate. The Centers for Disease Control and Prevention has been tracking these changes, as have other surveillance systems, such as the Autism and Developmental Disabilities Monitoring Network comprising 11 sites in the United States.[1] Another team of international researchers published their findings on the global prevalence of autism and other developmental disorders in 2012.[13]

Several factors seem to contribute to this increase in prevalence. Historically, in the 1960s and 1970s, the prevalence was low; this was during the time though when many individuals were identified with mental retardation (now known as intellectual disability) and were institutionalized. Once autism became a recognized diagnostic term in the 1980s, prevalence began to increase at the same time there was a decline in diagnosis of other disorders. The broadening of the diagnostic criteria seen with *DSM-III* and *-IV* further affected numbers. Direct testing for autism became available in 2001 with the Autism Diagnostic Observation Schedule (ADOS). The ADOS-2 with the Toddler Module was released in 2012, allowing for testing of children as young as 12 months old. Several experts in the field have participated in extensive research on the topic of rising prevalence of autism. **Box 1** highlights several contributors to increased prevalence, including an increase in diagnosis and shifting diagnostic criteria.[13,14]

AREAS OF VULNERABILITY
Comorbid Medical and Mental Health Conditions

It is estimated that more than 70% of individuals with autism have coexisting medical, developmental, and psychiatric conditions.[5] Gastrointestinal problems, sleep disorders, and epilepsy are the most common medical conditions. ADHD is one of the most common comorbid developmental conditions, which can significantly interfere with educational functioning. High activity, impulsivity, and easy distractibility make it harder for children to function in an integrated classroom. Recognizing signs and symptoms of ADHD early and providing diagnosis and treatment can contribute to improved functioning. Intellectual disability, another comorbid developmental

---

Box 1
Factors that may account for increase in prevalence of autism

1. Broadening of diagnostic criteria

2. Increased efficacy over time in case identification methods

3. Changes in diagnostic practices

4. Diagnostic substitution or switching

condition, impacts functioning and medical care. Some children are not able to use spoken language to communicate, which affects medical visits. For instance, this can impact a physician's ability to determine the source of pain or other medical conditions.

Mental health conditions further compound these difficulties. Social anxiety and generalized anxiety disorder are the most prevalent with rate estimates of 42% to 56%.[5] Even those who have strong language abilities may find it difficult to communicate in stressful situations, such as a medical setting. Children may not be able to identify as anxious, but they may present as irritable and angry. Although obsessive compulsive disorder (OCD) is also seen in children with ASD, it is important to recognize the difference between perseverating on topics of high interest common to autism, and intrusive disturbing anxiety-provoking thoughts that lead to compulsive behaviors more characteristic of OCD. Depression, which is also prevalent in this population, is more common in adults[5] (**Fig. 1**).

Sensory Processing Differences

Individuals with ASD have pronounced sensory difficulties to varying degrees. Tomchek and Dunn[4] found almost 100% of their sample reported sensory differences.

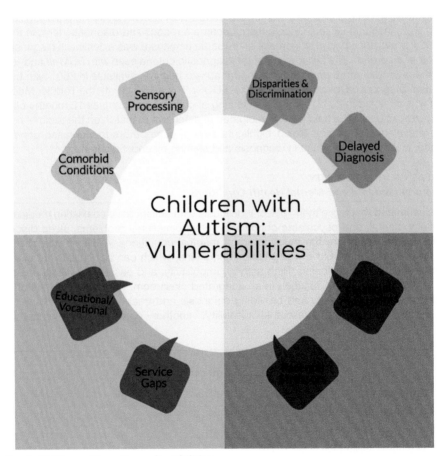

Fig. 1. Children with autism vulnerabilities.

Another study found abnormal auditory, visual, touch, and oral sensory processing that were significantly different from controls.[15] Individuals are often bothered by crowds or noise, bright lights and vivid colors, sudden changes, or surprises. They may have difficulty regulating responses and controlling impulses. They may engage in repetitive stereotyped behaviors as a form of self-calming. Behaviors can include hand flapping, rocking, pacing, quiet humming, or wiggling. When stressed, individuals have difficulty retrieving information and thinking clearly. They may have a low frustration tolerance, experience sensory overload, and become irritable, angry, and even aggressive. There is a higher incidence of aggressive behaviors often directed toward the caregiver and self-injurious behaviors that can occur when the person is stressed. These behaviors usually correlate with lower levels of speech and cognitive abilities.[6]

Barriers to Accessing Diagnostic and Therapeutic Services

There are several factors cited in studies to address the unequal access to autism diagnosis and treatment. Multiple studies revealed racial/ethnic disparities in diagnosis and treatment of children with ASD.[16–18] ASD care has also been found to differ by parental proficiency in English. For example, Latino children are less often diagnosed before age 4 compared with non-Latino children. After diagnosis, Latino children with ASD receive fewer evidence-based treatments and less medical specialty care than non-Latino white children.[2] Socioeconomic status has also been noted to influence services provided to children with ASD. Families with higher maternal education and knowledge about ASD care regardless of ethnicity are able to access more services.[2] Reasons for disparities include bias and lack of cultural training among providers, lack of information and knowledge about autism and treatment among families, language barriers, and limited resources to seek out and access the best services.[2] Oftentimes there is a lack of specialized diagnostic providers with long wait times for diagnosis and diagnostic services at specialty centers.

Finances Limit Access to Essential Interventions

Families of individuals who have ASD typically accrue higher medical expenses than families who are not caring for an individual with a developmental disability. Because of the nature of ASD, these individuals can require multiple therapies, including speech and language, feeding therapy, behavior therapy, occupational therapy, or physical therapy. Psychiatry and counseling are common medical supports used as well. These extensive therapies can also limit a parent's ability to work outside the home. Behavioral difficulties that lead to time out of school also interfere with caregiver work schedule, impacting finances.

Applied behavioral analysis (ABA) therapy, an evidenced-based therapy, is an integral component of an individual's and family's success throughout the lifetime of the patient. More specifically, using the processes of functional behavior assessment and functional analysis, the meaning behind the individual's behavior can be better understood so that the function of that behavior can be interpreted in order to guide the collaborative care team in knowing how to support the patient's medical experiences.[19] ABA therapy applies to all environments, situations, and experiences to which the individual is exposed across the lifespan.

Lack of adequate insurance creates a barrier to care. Coverage of ABA therapy varies by states. Medicaid, which is a main source of health care for low-income children, does not cover necessary ABA therapy in many states. Although private insurance often covers several hours of therapy a week, families may have cost-prohibitive deductibles or copays.

Family Stressors Contribute to Disparities in Health Care for Children with Autism Spectrum Disorder

Berg and colleagues[20] found that children with ASD had a significantly higher probability of having a greater number of Adverse Childhood Experiences (ACE) than those children without ASD. This increased experience of adversities potentially compromises chances for optimal physical and behavioral health outcomes. In a follow-up study, an association was found between increased ACEs and unmet health care needs in children with ASD. Poor parental health, residential instability, and economic hardship have been linked to gaps in insurance enrollment and lower use of preventative health care for children. This cross-sectional data analysis suggests psychosocial stressors may be a barrier to health care for children with ASD, specifically, medical, dental, and mental health services. This study also finds that care coordination was associated with a significantly lower number of unmet needs, highlighting the value of the medical home model.[21] Parents of children with ASD are at an increased risk of divorce.[22] Another study found the divorce rate among parents of children with ASD to be 6% higher than the national average.[23] ASD symptom severity also has been found to correlate to higher levels of maternal stress and psychopathology symptoms.[24]

Children with Autism Spectrum Disorder More Susceptible to Bullying, Discrimination, and Stereotyping

Recent findings show that children with ASD are bullied by their peers 3 to 4 times that of nondisabled peers.[7] Several studies have shown that the likelihood of being bullied increases in the context of exposure to certain risk factors, including behavioral difficulties and poor peer relationships.[8] Parents and school programs have been found to be able to modulate the negative impact of the victimization of bullying in children with ASD. One study found cyberbullying victimization was associated with peer rejection, anxiety, and depression in adolescents with ASD.[9]

Children with Autism Spectrum Disorder More Susceptible to Abuse

One population-based study found that children with ASD are more likely to be abused than those children with intellectual disability alone, and those children with both autism and intellectual disability are at greatest risk. Children who have more difficulties with hyperactivity, temper tantrums, and aggressions are most susceptible to maltreatment.[25]

Educational and Vocational Vulnerabilities

Children with ASD are particularly vulnerable at times of educational transition. Moving from the early intervention home-based program to special education preschool can lead to less intensive programming than the child had been receiving. Program decisions are at times based on a single observation, and individualized testing that may not provide a true sense of the child's level of functioning and impairment. Transition from preschool to elementary school can lead to declassification for some children with ASD when criteria for services are only based on academic functioning. Children who are in special education programs may not make adequate progress. One study found that individuals with autism were on average 4 years behind grade level in reading and almost 5 years behind in math, despite receiving high grades from teachers.[26] The discrepancy can lead to parental misperception about their child's abilities, contributing to unrealistic expectations. High-school programs often do not provide adequate vocational and adaptive skill development, and transition services can be limited, leaving adolescents ill prepared for the next stages of life.[10] As Bryna Siegel[27] discusses in her book, *The Politics of Autism*, inclusion is often promoted as an end rather than as a means, and it may not be appropriate for all children. Careful consideration needs to be given to individualized programming to meet the child's needs with monitoring to ensure progress. There is variation in educational programs and available vocational training depending on location. There is a role for the pediatrician to provide medical advocacy in the educational setting, writing prescriptions for ABA therapy and other needed therapies, reviewing educational testing with the family to ensure adequate progress, and assisting with transition into adulthood, emphasizing functional skill acquisition (**Box 2**).

THE ROLE OF THE PEDIATRICIAN

As the health care system moves toward a medical home model for improved care and prevention, primary pediatric providers are uniquely positioned as the first line of care for earlier identification of delays or indicators of ASD, referral for services, and full diagnostic evaluation.

There are indicators that children show signs of autism as early as 6 months of age.[28] Red flags include lack of response to name at 6 to 12 months, lack of pointing or gesturing to share interest, lack of single words. Formal screening for autism in the primary provider office is recommended by the American Academy of Pediatrics at 18 months and 24 months of age.[29] Moderate- to high-risk scores on screening warrant further evaluation by a specialist. There is no reason to wait and see how the child is progressing. Not only should the child be referred for full evaluation but also the primary provider can advocate for increased services while the child is waiting for diagnostic testing.

It is helpful for the primary provider who has a relationship with the family to begin the conversation about possible ASD. Providers need to be aware of their own perspective and possible implicit bias that they bring to the discussion. Physicians may be biased because of prior experience with complex patients. Any diagnosis that may involve learning disabilities or intellectual disability can be unconsciously viewed as particularly difficult for a family.[30] The bias not only applies to autism but also has been found to be particularly true for families of children with Down syndrome and other chromosomal differences. It may be helpful to view a diagnosis as unexpected news rather than bad news.

When beginning the conversation about possible autism with families, start with what the child can do. Point out the child's strengths and abilities. Provide hope with goals for the future. Be clear and say the word autism. When the primary provider partners with the specialist by laying out diagnostic possibilities, families have time to

---

Box 2
Educational advocacy from the medical provider

- Can keep the child on schedule for services
- Emphasize the need for appropriately intensive services
- Recommend consideration of inclusion in the least restrictive educational environment for academic challenges and peer modeling of typically developing children when possible and appropriate
- Assist the family in advocating at adolescent transition for appropriate functional skill development and vocational training
- Connect family to vocational rehabilitation counselors and advocates

prepare before their appointment with the specialist. Provide guidance for what the family can do immediately while waiting full diagnosis and offer resources to read. Plan for follow-up after the specialist appointment to reinforce diagnosis and support the family (**Box 3**).

Answering Common Questions Families Ask

Will my child be a fully functioning adult?

Research has demonstrated that early intensive intervention leads to improved outcomes.[3] A randomized controlled trial published in 2010 found increased IQ points, improved adaptive functioning, and increased likelihood to move along the autism spectrum continuum to the more mild end. There are misperceptions about intensive therapy for young children with ASD though. Families may be told that their child does not need intensive programming, ABA therapy is too harsh, or the child is not ready for intensive therapy. Medical advocacy is essential to reinforce the need for intensive services to optimize the child's functioning.

What more can a parent do to help the child?

Parents can be taught how to embed strategies to support social communication throughout everyday activities. One study found that children with individualized intensive parent training improved at a faster rate in daily living and social skills, suggesting the importance of parent coaching in natural environments.[31]

Did I cause this?

Even if parents do not ask, it is important to say to them, "You did not cause this." "It is not your fault." There is nothing that could have been done to prevent this. Consider the role of genetics and the need for further testing. Emphasize to families the current evidence about research showing no link between autism and vaccinations.[32]

Does my child have to be labeled?

It is essential to identify a child's strengths and challenges to provide targeted effective intervention. Diagnosis is often required to access autism-specific services through the school district and privately through insurance.

Is my child too young to be diagnosed?

Some children have clear symptoms of autism between 12 and 15 months of age that can be reliably diagnosed. The ADOS-2 Toddler Module can be administered between 12 and 30 months. One study compared children at 19 months and 36 months, finding stability of diagnosis over time. Children with ASD demonstrated improvement in social communication behaviors and an increase in repetitive behaviors as they got older.[33]

Box 3
Guiding families to move forward after diagnosis of autism spectrum disorder

Once the child has been diagnosed, the primary provider can provide the family 5 clear activities to do to proceed with care.
1. Contact early intervention to start or increase services.
2. Start or increase speech and language therapy to improve spontaneous functional communication.
3. Implement Applied Behavior Analysis to learn new skills, follow directions, and improve child's interactions.
4. Track child's progress.
5. If the child is approaching 3 years old, contact the school district for services.

How do I get my child into preschool?
The process for entry into special education preschool should begin when the child is approximately 2.5 years of age because it generally can take about 4 to 6 months from start to finish. The family needs to contact the school district in writing to request evaluation. They also need to register with the district. Once an evaluation has been requested, the district will meet with the family to determine further testing and program.

Does my child need medication?
Consider alpha-adrenergic agonists, clonidine or guanfacine, if needed for severe dysregulation, aggression, or safety concerns. Atypical antipsychotic medications, risperidone and aripiprazole, have been approved for use in children with autism for severe aggression and behavior problems.[34] Comorbid conditions, including ADHD and anxiety, may need medical treatment.

Are there any alternative medicines that we can use?
Higher rates of complementary alternative medicine (CAM) use have been found in children with classic autism, and children with coexisting conditions, including gastrointestinal symptoms, seizures, or evidence of behavior problems. Children taking psychotropic medications had lower use of special diets.[35] Most CAM treatments have not been adequately studied and do not have evidence to support their use.[36]

HELPING INDIVIDUALS WITH AUTISM SPECTRUM DISORDER NAVIGATE THE MEDICAL ENCOUNTER
Medical Home for Children with Autism Spectrum Disorder

The American Academy of Pediatrics developed the medical home as a model of delivering primary care that is accessible, continuous, comprehensive, family-centered, coordinated, compassionate, and culturally effective for every child and adolescent. Families of children with ASD were found to be less likely to receive care in a medical home compared with other children with special health care needs.[37–39]

It has been recommended by the American Academy of Pediatrics for medical homes to monitor the child's progress being made via related services being provided, educating families on appropriate evidence-based treatment models, linking them to a care coordinator, and proactively engaging them in a transition process between early intervention and preschool local services.[40] A care coordinator in the office provides essential supports and links for families throughout childhood and adolescence (**Box 4**).

MODELS FOR PREVENTION OR MANAGEMENT AND SYSTEMS OF CARE

A key component of the medical home is care coordination across settings and services (**Fig. 2**). For children with ASD and their families, this includes medical, educational, and behavioral team members. Care plans with an emphasis on goals with specific measures can lead to better outcomes. The American Academy of Pediatrics Policy Statement on patient and family-centered care coordination stresses the importance of patient and family-centered care that is planned, proactive, and comprehensive. It promotes self-care skills and independence. Electronic information technologies allow for increased ease of collaboration among caregivers, and parent portals allow families increased access to their medical information. Care coordination reimbursement codes can be used.[41]

Box 4
Role of care coordinator in primary medical provider setting

A designated staff member as care coordinator can
- Contact the family or individual in advance of appointments to determine any special needs.
- Arrange tour of office before first visit to encourage comfort and familiarity.
- Schedule appointment for first visit in AM or first afternoon slot to avoid crowds in the waiting room and extended wait time.
- Meet the family and individual upon arrival to the office to facilitate ease of visit.
- Notify physician and other staff of the individual's needs.
- Facilitate and coordinate appointments with other specialists.
- Coordinate with school district when necessary.
- Suggest family use social story before visit to describe the visit and what will occur.
- Provide sensory toys to child to assist with calming child to improve compliance.
- Use coping passport so the individual's medical and developmental profile is available for all care providers and specialists.

Transitioning Adolescence to Adulthood

Assisting the adolescent and family as they transition into adulthood involves more than just effectively transferring care to a physician for adults. This critical timeframe

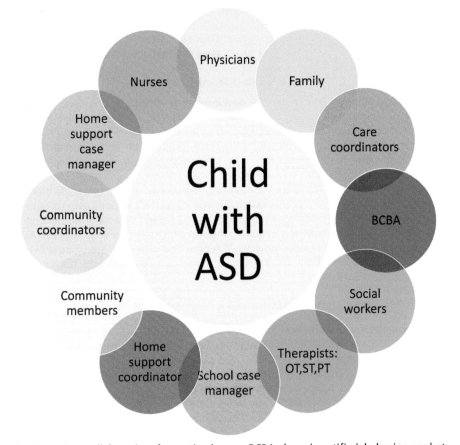

Fig. 2. Autism collaboration for optimal care. BCBA, board certified behavior analyst; OT, occupational therapist; PT, physical therapist; ST, speech therapist.

from 14 years to 21 years includes attention to medical and mental health issues; educational advocacy and vocational planning; navigating legal issues, such as obtaining guardianship or power of attorney and setting up trusts; and accessing appropriate community agencies: Division of Developmental Disability as needed, Association of Retarded Citizens, Supplemental Security Income/Medicaid, and autism support agencies.

The American Academy of Pediatrics clinical report on health care transitions provides guidelines for transitioning all adolescents.[42] One study found that only 21% of adolescents with ASD receive any transition planning services.[43] Of those pediatric providers with extensive experience caring for youth with ASD, 5 interventions were identified. These interventions include the following: (1) Write medical summary to give to adult physician, (2) Provide family with list of available adult providers, (3) Coordinate care and communication between pediatric and adult physicians, (4) Schedule a transition-specific appointment to discuss the issues with the individual and family, and (5) Use checklist to track transition progress.[43]

ROLE OF TECHNOLOGY IN CAUSING OR MANAGING THE ISSUES

The use of technology in intervention and instruction for children and adolescents with ASD is increasing at a striking rate. Children with ASD often use educational and recreational apps at home and school to promote learning and for communication. Children with ASD seem to have an affinity for using technologies, such as smart phones and tablets. The use of portable tablet computers and multimedia players as a speech-generating device has an emerging evidence base.[44] Social

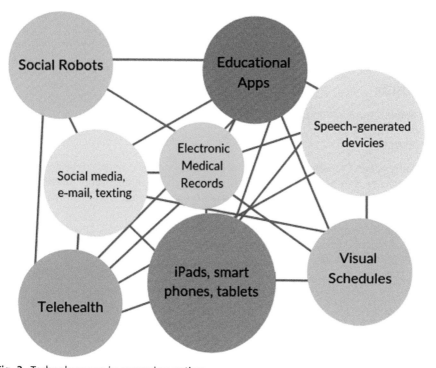

Fig. 3. Technology use in managing autism.

robots are being increasingly used to enhance social skills and communication. Robots have been shown to have social and behavioral benefits for children with ASD, including heightened engagement, increased attention, and decreased social anxiety.[45] High-school students with ASD reported that the use of technology in school and home settings helped them to improve their independence, reduce their anxiety, and increase their social opportunities.[46] Social media, e-mail, and texting can expand opportunities for social interactions. Technology can provide opportunities to develop social and technical skills needed later for employment (**Fig. 3**).

Telehealth uses technology for remote training and supervision. It provides opportunities as an innovative model for service delivery of behavioral interventions, especially because of the shortage of highly qualified professionals to adequately meet the needs and demands in this area.

Digital media is an area of high interest for some children and adolescents with ASD. Although it can be an excellent teaching tool, there is the hazard of Internet overuse and electronic addiction.

SUMMARY

Autism is a lifelong disorder, but there is a vast range of levels of functioning and need for supports. Early diagnosis of ASDs with intensive targeted intervention has the potential to greatly improve functioning. There are many barriers to optimal care though. Regardless of an autism diagnosis, the whole child needs to be treated, assessing and building on strengths while intervening for weaknesses that are maladaptive and interfere with functioning. Using the team approach both in the office and in the community is essential ongoing management for children with autism and their families. Medical, behavioral, and educational services need to be linked and provided collaboratively. Although there have been improvements in the care of this population, much still needs to be done to continue to address ongoing needs particularly for individuals entering adulthood.

DISCLOSURE

The authors have nothing to disclose.

REFERENCES

1. Christensen DL, Braun KV, Baio J, et al. Prevalence and characteristics of autism spectrum disorder among children aged 8 years—autism and developmental disabilities monitoring network, 11 sites, United States, 2012. MMWR Surveill Summ 2018;65(13):1.

2. Magana S, Lopez K, Aguinaga A, et al. Access to diagnosis and treatment services among Latino children with autism spectrum disorders. Intellect Dev Disabil 2013;51(3):141–53.

3. Dawson G, Rogers S, Munson J, et al. Randomized, controlled trial of an intervention for toddlers with autism: the Early Start Denver model. Pediatrics 2010; 125(1):e17–23.

4. Tomchek SD, Dunn W. Sensory processing in children with and without autism: a comparative study using the short sensory profile. Am J Occup Ther 2007;61(2): 190–200.

5. Lai MC, Lombardo M, Baron-Cohen S. Autism. Lancet 2014;383:896–910.

6. Fitzpatrick S, Srivorakiat L, Erickson C, Wink L, et al. Aggression in autism spectrum disorder: presentation and treatment options. Neuropsychiatr Dis Treat 2016;12:1525–38.

7. Hoover DW, Kaufman J. Adverse childhood experiences in children with autism spectrum disorder. Curr Opin Psychiatry 2018;31(2):128–32.

8. Hebron J, Oldfield J, Humphrey N. Cumulative risk effects in the bullying of children and young people with autism spectrum conditions. Autism 2017;21(3):291–300.

9. Wright MF, Wachs S. Does peer rejection moderate the associations among cyberbullying victimization, depression, and anxiety among adolescents with autism spectrum disorder? Children 2019;6(3):41.

10. Friedman ND, Warfield ME, Parish SL. Transition to adulthood for individuals with autism spectrum disorder: current issues and future perspectives. Neuropsychiatry 2013;3(2):181.

11. Wehmeyer ML. The story of intellectual disability: an evolution of meaning, understanding, and public perception. Baltimore (MD): Brookes Publishing Co.; 2013.

12. Volkmar FR, Reichow B. Autism in DSM-5: progress and challenges. Mol Autism 2013;4:13.

13. Elsabbagh M, Divan G, Koh Y-J, et al. Global prevalence of autism and other pervasive developmental disorders. Autism Res 2012;5(3):160–79.

14. Fombonne E. Editorial: the rising prevalence of autism. J Child Psychol Psychiatry 2018;59(7):717–20.

15. Kern JK, Trivedi MH, Garver CR, et al. The pattern of sensory processing abnormalities in autism. Autism 2006;10(5):480–94.

16. Corcoran J, Berry A, Hill S. The lived experience of US parents of children with autism spectrum disorders. J Intellect Disabil 2015;19(4):356–66.

17. Durkin MS, Maenner MJ, Baio J, et al. Autism spectrum disorder among US children (2002–2010): socioeconomic, racial, and ethnic disparities. Am J Public Health 2017;107(11):1818–26.

18. Broder-Fingert S, Shui A, Pulcini CD, et al. Racial and ethnic differences in subspecialty service use by children with autism. Pediatrics 2013;132(1):94–100.

19. Iwata BA, Dozier CL. Clinical application of functional analysis methodology. Behav Anal Pract 2008;1(1):3–9.

20. Berg KL, Shiu CS, Acharya K, et al. Disparities in adversity among children with autism spectrum disorder: a population-based study. Dev Med Child Neurol 2016;58(11):1124–31.

21. Berg KL, Shiu C-S, Feinstein RT, et al. Adverse childhood experiences are associated with unmet healthcare needs among children with autism spectrum disorder. J Pediatr 2018;202:258–64.

22. Hartley S, Barker E, Seitger M, et al. The relative risk and timing of divorce in families of children with an autism spectrum disorder. J Fam Psychol 2010;24(4):449–57.

23. Risdal D, Singer G. Marital advancement in parents of children with disabilities: a historical review and meta-analysis. Res Pract Persons Disabilities 2004;29(2):45–103.

24. Tomeny TS. Parenting stress as an indirect pathway to mental health concerns among mothers of children with autism spectrum disorder. Autism 2017;21(7):907–11.

25. Mcdonnell CG, Boan AD, Bradley CC, et al. Child maltreatment in autism spectrum disorder and intellectual disability: results from a population-based sample. J Child Psychol Psychiatry 2018;60(5):576–84.

26. Wagner M, Marder C, Blackorby J, et al. The achievements of youth with disabilities during secondary school. Menlo Park (CA): SRI International; 2003.

27. Siegel B. The politics of autism. Oxford (United Kingdom): Oxford University Press, Incorporated; 2018.

28. Nadig AS, Ozonoff S, Young GS, et al. A prospective study of response to name in infants at risk for autism. Arch Pediatr Adolesc Med 2007;161(4):378–83.

29. Zwaigenbaum L, Bauman ML, Fein D, et al. Early screening of autism spectrum disorder: recommendations for practice and research. Pediatrics 2015; 136(Supplement 1):S41–59.

30. Carroll C, Carroll C, Goloff N, et al. When bad news isn't necessarily bad: recognizing provider bias when sharing unexpected news. Pediatrics 2018; 142(1):7–10.

31. Wetherby AM, Guthrie W, Woods J, et al. Parent-implemented social intervention for toddlers with autism: an RCT. Pediatrics 2014;134(6):1084–93.

32. Maglione M, Das L, Raaen L, et al. Safety of vaccines used for routine immunizations of US children. Pediatrics 2014;134:325–37.

33. Guthrie W, Swineford LB, Nottke C, et al. Early diagnosis of autism spectrum disorder: stability and change in clinical diagnosis and symptom presentation. J Child Psychol Psychiatry 2012;54(5):582–90.

34. Fung LK, Mahajan R, Nozzolillo A, et al. Pharmacologic treatment of severe irritability and problem behaviors in autism: a systematic review and meta-analysis. Pediatrics 2016;137(Supplement):124–35.

35. Perrin JM, Coury DL, Hyman SL, et al. Complementary and alternative medicine use in a large pediatric autism sample. Pediatrics 2012;130(Supplement 2).

36. Levy SE, Hyman SL. Complementary and alternative medicine treatments for children with autism spectrum disorders. Child Adolesc Psychiatr Clin N Am 2008; 17(4):803–20.

37. Hyman SL, Johnson JK. Autism and pediatric practice: toward a medical home. J Autism Dev Disord 2012;42(6):1156–64.

38. Liptak GS, Orlando M, Yingling JT, et al. Satisfaction with primary health care received by families of children with developmental disabilities. J Pediatr Health Care 2006;20(4):245–52.

39. Carbone PS, Behl DD, Azor V, et al. The medical home for children with autism spectrum disorders: parent and pediatrician perspectives. J Autism Dev Disord 2009;40(3):317–24.

40. Adams RC, Tapia C. Early intervention, IDEA Part C services, and the medical home: collaboration for best practice and best outcomes. Pediatrics 2013; 132(4):e1073–88.

41. Council on Children with Disabilities and Medical Home Implementation Project Advisory Committee. Patient and family centered care coordination: a framework for integrating care for children and youth across multiple systems (Policy statement). Pediatrics 2014;133(5):e1451–60.

42. White PH, Cooley WC, Transitions Clinical Report Authoring Group; American Academy of Pediatrics; American Academy of Family Physicians; American College of Physicians. Supporting the health care transition from adolescence to adulthood in the medical home. Pediatrics 2018;142(5):e20182587. Pediatrics. 2019;143(2).

43. Kuhlthau KA, Warfield ME, Hurson J, et al. Pediatric provider's perspectives on the transition to adult health care for youth with autism spectrum disorder: current strategies and promising new directions. Autism 2014;19(3):262–71.

44. Lorah E, Parnell A, Schaefer P, et al. A systematic review of tablet computers and portable media players as speech generating devices for individuals with autism spectrum disorder. J Autism Dev Disord 2015;45:3792–804.
45. Sartorato F, Przybylowski L, Sarko D. Improving therapeutic customs in autism spectrum disorders: enhancing social communication and sensory processing through the use of interactive robots. J Psychiatr Res 2017;90:1–11.
46. Hedges SH, Odom SL, Hume K, et al. Technology use as a support tool by secondary students with autism. Autism 2017;22(1):70–9.

Homelessness in Pediatric Populations

Strategies for Prevention, Assistance, and Advocacy

Meera S. Beharry, MD, FSAHM[a,b],*, Randal Christensen, MD, MPH[c]

KEYWORDS

- Homeless • Experiencing homelessness • Pediatric • Children • Adolescent
- Youth • Runaway • Trafficking

KEY POINTS

- Children and adolescents experience homelessness at higher rates than point-in-time counts suggest.
- Many pediatricians see patients and their families who are unstably housed or homeless without being aware of their status.
- Through increased awareness of the health issues facing pediatric patients experiencing homelessness, pediatricians can identify those at risk and provide links to needed care and support services.
- This article reviews current data about homelessness among pediatric populations in the United States and strategies for intervention.

INTRODUCTION

Homelessness dramatically increases morbidity and mortality. Health issues also increase the likelihood of families experiencing homelessness.[1] Pediatricians have a unique opportunity to prevent and intervene in pediatric and family homelessness[2] because they are well versed in assessing social determinants of health, providing anticipatory guidance and working with schools and other community partners. This article provides an overview of health issues facing pediatric patients and their families when experiencing homelessness, ideas for identifying families who are currently

---

[a] Adolescent Medicine, McLane Children's Medical Center, McLane Children's Specialty Clinic, Baylor Scott and White, 1901 SW H.K. Dodgen Loop, MS-CK-300, Building 300, Temple, TX 76502, USA; [b] Texas A&M Health Science Center (Affiliate), Temple, TX, USA; [c] Randal Christensen Consulting, LLC, 2654 W Horizon Ridge Parkway Suite B5-113, Henderson, NV 89052, USA
* Corresponding author.
E-mail address: Meera.Beharry@BSWHealth.org
Twitter: @mbeharrymd (M.S.B.); @AskMeWhyIHurt (R.C.)

Pediatr Clin N Am 67 (2020) 357–372
https://doi.org/10.1016/j.pcl.2019.12.007
0031-3955/20/© 2019 Elsevier Inc. All rights reserved.

experiencing homelessness as well as those at risk of becoming homeless. This article also suggests areas for advocacy and provides strategies for pediatricians to intervene, and ultimately, prevent homelessness.

BACKGROUND

There have been 2 notable periods of mass homelessness: The Great Depression and the period from the 1980s to 2019.[3] The current wave of mass homelessness is, at least in part, attributed to the inadequacy of mainstream safety net programs to meet the high level of need. Programs, such as Medicaid, Temporary Assistance to Needy Families (TANF), and Supplemental Nutrition Assistance Program (SNAP, formerly food stamps), have had funding restrictions and increased documentation requirements, which have made them inaccessible for many families.[3]

The Stewart B. McKinney Homeless Assistance Act of 1987 was initially introduced to Congress in 1986 as the Homeless Person's Survival Act. On Oct 30, 2000, the legislation was renamed as the McKinney-Vento Homeless Assistance Act after the death of one of its lead supporters, Representative Bruce Vento.[4] This landmark legislation provided a clear definition of homelessness and areas for intervention.

Presently, there are several definitions of homelessness.[5] In the Runaway and Homeless Youth Act, a homeless youth is someone who is "not more than 21 years of age...for whom it is not possible to live in a safe environment with a relative and who have no other safe alternative living arrangement."[5,6] The Homeless Emergency Assistance and Rapid Transition to Housing (HEARTH) Act of 2009 consolidated 3 different programs under the McKinney-Vento Homeless Assistance Act into a single grant program in addition to revising and renaming Emergency Shelter programs and grants and creating the Rural Housing Stability program. The HEARTH Act definition includes the following 4 categories for homelessness:

1. "Individuals and families who lack a fixed, regular, and adequate nighttime residence and includes a subset for an individual who resided in an emergency shelter or a place not meant for human habitation and who is exiting an institution where he or she temporarily resided;
2. Individuals and families who will imminently lose their primary nighttime residence;
3. Unaccompanied youth and families with children and youth who are defined as homeless under other federal statutes who do not otherwise qualify as homeless under this definition;
4. Individuals and families who are fleeing, or are attempting to flee, domestic violence, dating violence, sexual assault, stalking, or other dangerous or life-threatening conditions that relate to violence against the individual or a family member."[7]

For homeless families, episodes of homelessness are part of a cycle of housing instability precipitated by living in deep poverty; lack of available, affordable, and safe housing; and "doubling-up," that is, living with family and friends in overcrowded settings to reduce financial stress. Before the first episode of homelessness, families are likely to have already been receiving services from safety net programs, such as Medicaid and SNAP, but an acute increase in financial or social stress disrupts the fragile balance. Severe illness, loss of a job, or change in family dynamics owing to incarceration, involvement with child protection services, or domestic violence is a common precipitating factor.[8]

Youth homelessness can be temporary or cyclic. As noted by Auerswald and Eyre,[9] there are definable phases of a youth's experience of homelessness when they are more likely to leave or return to the streets. Youth are more likely to access health services during the "extrication" phase and more likely to access substance use treatment during the "disequilibrium" phase[10] (**Fig. 1**).

EPIDEMIOLOGY

Data estimating the number of people experiencing homelessness are inherently limited by several factors, including variable definitions of homelessness and lack of fixed contact points for the study population.[11] These limitations result lead to oversampling of those in shelter; however, the number of shelters is very limited even in the largest cities. Many shelters do not take residents who are not part of what has been previously described as "traditional families," for example, gay parents, a single father with children; families with older teens, pregnant teens, or those suffering substance abuse or severe mental health problems. When counting homeless youth, there are additional challenges related to youth avoiding formal systems of shelter because of stigma, fear of legal action, or fear of being returned to abusive situations.[11–13]

The primary reference used to estimate the population of people experiencing homelessness in America is the point-in-time count, which is usually conducted on 1 night in January.[14] Data from the 2018 point-in-time count indicate that there were roughly 553,000 people experiencing homelessness in the United States, approximately two-thirds of whom were in shelter. For the point-in-time count, "people in families with children" are defined as "people who are homeless as part of a household that has at least one adult (age 18 or older) and one child under age 18." More than 180,000 of the approximately half a million people experiencing homelessness are people in families with children.[14] Data from previous point-in-time counts show that more than 75% of the adults in homeless families are women and that the adults in homeless families tend to be younger, between the ages of 18 and 30. Furthermore, 59% of people experiencing homelessness in families were children under age 18; almost half of these children were under age 6, and 10% were under 1 year old. "The age at which a person in the United States is most likely to stay in a homeless shelter is infancy (**Fig. 2**)."[7,15]

Approximately 36,000 people in the 2018 point-in-time count were "unaccompanied youth": people under age 25 experiencing homelessness away from their family. An overwhelming majority (89%) of these youth were "transition age youth" (TAY) between the ages of 18 and 24. More than half of the unaccompanied youth were unsheltered, which is significantly higher than the rest of the counted population.[14]

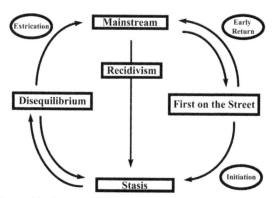

Fig. 1. The lifecycle model of youth homelessness. (*From* Auerswald CL, Eyre SL. Youth homelessness in San Francisco: a life cycle approach. Soc Sci Med. 2002 May;54(10):1497-512; with permission.)

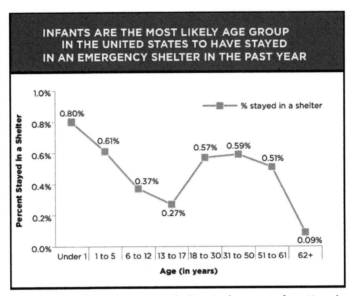

Fig. 2. Numbers experiencing an emergency shelter stay by age are from Homeless Management Information System Estimates for the 2013 Annual Homeless Assessment Report to Congress. (*From* Brown SR, Shinn M, Khadduri J. Homeless Families Research Brief: Well-being of Young Children After Experiencing Homelessness. Available at: https://www.acf.hhs.gov/sites/default/files/opre/opre_homefam_brief3_hhs_children_02_24_2017_b508.pdf.)

In an attempt to more accurately identify the population of homeless youth, Morton and colleagues[16] used a nationally representative phone-based survey to define the population of youth who have a variety of homeless experiences, including those who were "couch-surfing," that is, staying temporarily with friends or extended family members, in addition to those who met the traditional definitions of homelessness. Their data estimate that at least 660,000 youth aged 13 to 17 and 2.4 million youth aged 18 to 25 experienced at least 1 night of homelessness in 12 months before the study. In addition, there were no significant differences between those in rural versus nonrural counties. Youth who reported being unmarried with children of their own; lesbian, gay, bisexual, or transgender; black or African American; having not completed high school or passed a GED (General Educational Development) test; or with an annual household income of less than $24,000 were more likely to experience homelessness.

Data from the US Department of Education are congruent with those from the phone study indicating that more than 1.3 million children experiencing homelessness were enrolled in school for the 2016 to 2017 academic year. Of these students, almost a quarter million had disabilities, more than 118,000 were unaccompanied/living apart from their parents or guardians, and 16,170 were in migrant families. More than 75% of the 1.3 million children who were enrolled in public school and experiencing homelessness were "doubled up"; 3.7% were living in motels or hotels; 13.9% were living in shelters, transitional housing, or awaiting foster care placement; and 6.6% were unsheltered[17] (**Fig. 3**).

Youth who have been involved with the foster care system or who have been incarcerated are significantly more likely to experience prolonged youth homelessness. Prolonged youth homelessness is an umbrella term combining chronic homelessness,

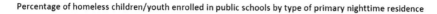

Percentage of homeless children/youth enrolled in public schools by type of primary nighttime residence

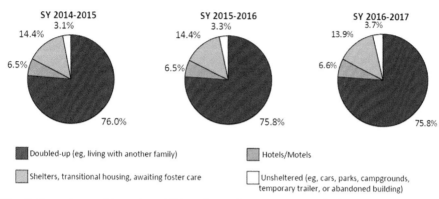

Fig. 3. Percentage of homeless children in grades pre-K-12 enrolled in public schools in the United States by type of primary nighttime residence. (*From* National Center for Homeless Education. National Overview. Available at: http://profiles.nche.seiservices.com/ConsolidatedStateProfile.aspx.)

which is 12 or more months of homelessness, and long-term homelessness, experiencing homelessness for at least 5 years.[18] In a study of TAY in Los Angeles, Rice[19] found that more than 61% of participants who had been incarcerated before age 18 experienced long-term homelessness.

According to the "Trafficking in Persons Report," "severe forms of trafficking in persons" is defined as "sex trafficking in which a commercial sex act is induced by force, fraud, or coercion, or in which the person induced to perform such an act has not attained 18 years of age; or the recruitment, harboring, transportation, provision, or obtaining of a person for labor or services, through the use of force, fraud, or coercion for the purpose of subjection to involuntary servitude, peonage, debt bondage, or slavery." The report states "in the United States, traffickers prey upon children in the foster care system."[20] The enactment of the Justice for Victims of Trafficking Act in 2015 required states to change their laws to include any finding of commercial sexual exploitation (CSE) involving a minor to automatically meet criteria for child abuse and neglect.[21]

HEALTH ISSUES

The issues of data accuracy in defining and counting the number of children experiencing homelessness extend to data regarding the incidence and prevalence of health conditions. Generally, most studies use the McKinney-Vento or HEARTH definitions of homelessness because recruitment is conducted at sites that use these definitions to assess eligibility for services. It is clear those experiencing homelessness are significantly more likely to have poor health and experience more adverse childhood events than those who are stably housed.[2,22–25]

Physical Health

Infancy
A multistate study conducted from 2009 to 2015 found that children born to caregivers (parent answering the survey) who were homeless "prenatally and postnatally," or who were homeless "postnatally only" were significantly more likely to have a postnatal hospitalization, be described as having "fair or poor health" and to be at

developmental risk compared with those whose caregivers were never homeless. Those who were homeless "prenatally only" did not have the increased developmental risk, but they still had higher risks of hospitalization and poorer health compared with the never homeless group. In addition, infants who had been homeless for more than 6 months were more likely to have an overweight status in addition to the higher risks of hospitalization, poorer health, and developmental risks.[25]

Asthma

Because of issues related to poor housing or being unsheltered, children and youth experiencing homelessness are more likely to experience exacerbations of asthma than housed youth. In 1 analysis of more than 70,000 pediatric asthma hospitalizations in New York State, youth who were identified as homeless were more than 31 times more likely to be admitted than those who were not homeless. The homeless subgroup was more likely to have been admitted from the emergency department and those older than 5 years old were more likely to require ventilation than patients older than 5 years old who were not homeless.[26]

Obesity/malnutrition

The relationship between food insecurity, socioeconomic status, and obesity is complex. For many people with limited resources, inexpensive, low-nutrient, high-calorie foods are more easily available than more nutritious options.[27–29] Many shelters, drop-ins, and soup kitchens serve processed foods. People who are living in hotels, in cars, or on the streets will not have access to refrigerators and cooking facilities. Those who are doubled up may have limited access to shared kitchen space. Fast food becomes the most available option. In a study of children accessing care through New York Children's Health Project, which provides comprehensive primary health care to homeless children and families via mobile and on-site clinics at family shelters, domestic violence shelters, and a shelter for homeless youth, 39% of the children met definitions of overweight or obese.[27] Compounding the problem for children is the lack of safe places to engage in physical activity or play.[28]

Dental problems

Dental problems are common for many children, but particular challenges exist for those who are homeless.[30,31] Children experiencing homelessness generally lack access to the basic tools needed for dental care, such as toothbrushes, toothpaste, and access to clean water.[30] In their study of youth aged 14 to 28 who identified as homeless and were accessing care at a community health center in Seattle, Chi and Milgrom[30] found that approximately one-third of youth surveyed reported their oral health as "very bad" or "bad" and had problems such as sensitive teeth, discolored teeth, toothaches, broken fillings or teeth, sore or bleeding gums, pain while chewing, a loose tooth, poorly fitting dental repairs, or tooth abscess. Obviously, these dental problems can affect nutritional intake and other aspects of health.

Vision problems

Vision problems are common among pediatric patients experiencing homelessness.[32,33] Estimates of vision problems range between 13% to 26% of those studied.[33] Using a combination of the vision screening with a questionnaire developed in accordance with the American Academy of Pediatrics and Ophthalmology Policy Statement on "Eye Examination in Infants, Children and Young Adults by Pediatricians," eye-chart screening and referral to ophthalmologic examination for those who failed screening, Smith and colleagues[33] found a prevalence of vision problems of 25%. Myopia and astigmatism were the most common problems, but the ophthalmologic examination revealed additional diagnoses of amblyopia, anisome-tropia, esotropia, hyperopia, myopia, nystagmus, and ocular albinism. Getting new glasses, or being able to replace or repair broken or lost glasses, is a significant challenge for many people experiencing homelessness because of insurance restrictions, lack of insurance, and limited availability of ophthalmology or resources to pay for glasses.[33]

Injury

Injuries are common because of the unsafe living situations of children and youth while homeless, trauma, and substance use. Injury was part of the diagnoses for approximately one-third of adolescents and young adults who used the emergency department or were admitted for inpatient care in a recent Seattle-based study of patients aged 15 to 25 who were admitted to the emergency department or inpatient floors and whose address was listed as "homeless," "none," a homeless shelter, or a service agency.[34]

Infection

Overcrowded conditions can also increase the risks of infection. There have been recent outbreaks of isoniazid-resistant tuberculosis among residents of homeless shelters in 16 states.[35] Outbreaks of hepatitis A, head lice, and body lice with associated *Bartonella quintana* have occurred among homeless populations in the United States in recent years.[36,37] Homelessness was recently reported as a risk factor for adult admissions and readmissions for respiratory syncytial virus in Seattle.[38] There are obvious implications for children exposed to adults with these infections.

Scabies is more common among those who are homeless or unstably housed with a prevalence of 10% compared with a prevalence of less than 1% among children seen in routine primary care practices. In addition, more frequent episodes of common pediatric conditions, such as otitis media and gastroenteritis, occur among children experiencing homelessness.[22]

Sexually transmitted infections

Caccamo and colleagues[39] sought to estimate the prevalence of sexually transmitted infections (STIs) among youth experiencing homelessness by reviewing published studies from 2000 to 2015. They found that rates of chlamydia ranged from 4.2% to 11.6% in studies that relied on tested samples compared with 2.8% to 18.3% that relied on self-reported diagnosis. Gonorrhea prevalence from tested samples was 0.4% to 11% and from 1.0% to 24.9% from self-report. Prevalence of syphilis was 0.2% to 3.5%, and 1.1% to 11.8% for prevalence of herpes. There were only 3 articles reporting the prevalence of hepatitis B with rates ranging from 1.4% to 17%. The 2 articles reporting on hepatitis C noted a prevalence of 3.7% to 12%. Medlow and colleagues[40] found variability in rates of human immunodeficiency virus in studies of homeless youth in the United States ranging from 2.3% to 13.6%.

Not surprisingly, rates are higher among youth with a history of being victims of human trafficking or CSE. Recent studies of populations who experienced CSE found 21% to 37% were positive for STIs.[21,41]

Pregnancy

An adolescent pregnancy may be the cause of homelessness for some youth or a result. An analysis of the National Longitudinal Study of Adolescent Health found that girls who ran away in the past year had over twice the risk of pregnancy compared with those who did not. These risks were higher for those who had been victims of sexual assault or those who identified as racial minorities.[42] An analysis from the Runaway/Homeless

Youth Management Information System supported the findings of higher risks of pregnancy among those who identified as African American or Hispanic.[43] Pregnant youth had higher rates of STIs, history of probation or felony charges, and history of emotional abuse by their mothers compared with nonpregnant homeless youth.[43] In their study of adolescent mothers who were homeless, Crawford and colleagues[44] found that approximately 56% had constant custody of their children and approximately 19% never had custody. Adolescents who have been pregnant and homeless have higher rates of mental health problems, such as major depression, posttraumatic stress disorder (PTSD), substance abuse, and antisocial personality disorder.[44]

Mental Health

As with other health issues, studies of the prevalence of mental health conditions among homeless youth are limited.[40] Many youth meet criteria for more than 1 mental health condition.[45]

Post-traumatic stress disorder

PTSD prevalence among adolescents has been estimated at 2% to 6% in community samples and 12% to 15% in those with a trauma history. Among youth who had experienced trauma once on the streets, the prevalence of PTSD was 17.7%.[46] Female adolescents or youth who identify as sexual minority youth are more likely to meet criteria PTSD.[40,45]

Depression/suicide

At least one-third and up to approximately one-half of homeless youth meet criteria for depression.[40] In their study of homeless families, Barnes and colleagues[47] found that youth in families experiencing homelessness were twice as likely to report self-injurious behavior and suicidal ideation, and 3 times as likely to report suicide attempts compared with their nonhomeless peers.[47]

Substance use

Substance use is a common problem among homeless youth. In a study of homeless youth aged 13 to 19, Ginzler and colleagues[48] found more than 94% used tobacco, alcohol, or marijuana in the past year, and 23% to 73% reported using other substances, such as quaaludes "downers", cocaine, heroin, amphetamines, and hallucinogens. Of the sample, approximately 86% met diagnostic criteria for dependence or abuse. In a study of youth experiencing homelessness in 7 states, 20% reported nonmedical use of prescription drugs.[49]

ACADEMIC PROBLEMS LEARNING DISABILITIES

As noted by Barnes and colleagues,[32] poor health is correlated with problems in executive functioning and some aspects of self-regulation, such as inhibitory or emotional control. Twenty months after an emergency shelter stay, children aged 18 to 41 months had higher risks of developmental delays and behavioral challenges and were disadvantaged in readiness for reading and math compared with their peers in national samples.[15] Of the more than 1.3 million homeless children and youth in school, almost a quarter million met criteria for a disability according to the Individuals with Disabilities Act.[17]

Frequent moves impact the ability to have consistent educational experiences and achievements.[2,50] Children and youth experiencing homelessness may come to school with little or no sleep or food. Those who are interested in participating in extracurricular activities may not be able to do so because they need to return to shelter or do not have the resources to participate. Although the McKinney-Vento legislation and Every Student Succeeds Act have provisions to allow students to stay at their previous school and to help with costs for participating in extracurricular activities, children or their guardians may not be aware of this.

ROLE OF THE PEDIATRICIAN/PUBLIC HEALTH ADVOCATE

The reader will note the use of the phrase "experiencing homelessness" rather than stating homeless children or homeless youth. Stigma associated with homelessness limits many people, but particularly children and adolescents from accessing services.[24] In addition, many adolescents or families might not consider themselves homeless when they are "couch-surfing" or doubled up.

Identifying At-Risk Families

Providing quality health care is a team sport. Front desk staff, medical assistants, and nurses may notice that a family's contact information has changed often. They may recognize the provided address as the address of a shelter. Some of the staff may also hear conversations about the patient's financial or housing situation that can indicate risk. They should be encouraged to respectfully share this information with clinicians and social work in a confidential setting.

Screening all patients and families for social and financial difficulties is 1 way to identify families who are already homeless as well as those at risk of homelessness. Prefacing questions with a statement about the relationship of housing and other social issues to health can help patients and their families understand that a pediatrician's motivation is to help them address all aspects of their health and well-being.

The following list provides suggestions for assessment questions:

For parents and guardians of younger children[51]

- What type of housing does the child live in?
- During the last 12 months, was there a time when you were not able to pay the mortgage or rent on time?
- In the past 12 months, how many places has the child lived?
- Since the child was born, has the child ever been homeless or lived in a shelter?

Other questions that were developed from the US Department of Housing and Urban Development, Health and Human Services, and Veterans Administration include the following[52]:

In the last 60 days, have you

- Been concerned about losing your housing
- Changed residences more than twice
- Lived with a friend or family member you do not normally reside with due to financial hardship
- Been evicted or served an eviction notice
- Slept outside, in an abandoned building, in your car, in an emergency shelter, or in a motel due to financial hardship?

For older children, adolescents, and young adults, in addition to asking about who lives at home and the safety of the home environment when speaking to the adolescent alone, providers can ask, "Have you ever seriously thought about running away from home?" If the young person answers "yes," asking where they would go and why they thought running away can help identify those at risk. Another follow-up question is, "Have you ever run away from home?," if they do not volunteer this information.

Taking a sexual history is a key part of the adolescent psychosocial assessment. In addition to the typical HEADSS assessment,[53] the following questions can be used to screen for CSE[54]:

- Have you ever had to have sex in exchange for something you wanted or needed (money, food, shelter, or other items)?
- Has anyone ever asked you to have sex with another person?

Prevention

All health care providers should be familiar with available resources for assisting homeless children and their families. Collaboration with social work, community health workers, and legal services is essential to identifying, assisting, and advocating for those experiencing homelessness. Because people experiencing homelessness have likely also had adverse childhood experiences (physical, emotional, or sexual abuse; physical or emotional neglect; household dysfunction: divorce, mental illness of a parent or guardian, witnessing domestic violence, incarcerated relative, or parental substance abuse) or other trauma, the authors recommend a strengths-based, resilience-building approach and trauma-informed approach to care.[24]

Food, Clothing, Shelter

In addition to helping patients and their families apply for Women, Infants, and Children (WIC) and SNAP, clinic staff can maintain lists of food banks, soup kitchens, and programs that will provide lunch in the summer for children who receive free or reduced lunch during the school years.[2] Educational interventions in shelters can help improve the variety and nutritional value of foods that children and youth eat.[27]

Some clinics, emergency departments, and hospitals will keep extra clothes for families to take if their clothes were ruined while seeking care. Local shelters and drop-in centers often receive donations for youth to choose from. Many drop-in centers for youth will have laundry services.

Many clinical settings include posters and information about domestic violence shelters, youth shelters, and/or the trafficking hotline number in the examination rooms or bathrooms. To help ensure safety, the authors recommend asking the patient if they might be hurt if they were found to have brochures or handouts with information about shelters and hotlines.

National Runaway Safeline: "The mission of the National Runaway Safeline is to keep America's runaway, homeless and at-risk youth safe and off the streets."

1-800-RUNAWAY
https://www.1800runaway.org/resources-links/

National Safe Place: Sites go through training to provide connection to emergency shelter. Many institutions, such as fire stations, city halls, bus lines, hospitals, and clinics, have become safe places. Teens can text for help or go to any facility with the national safe place logo for assistance.

https://www.nationalsafeplace.org/

Including the following information in patient handouts may be beneficial:

TXT 4 HELP is a nationwide, 24-hour text-for-support service for teens in crisis.
If you're in trouble or need help, text SAFE and your current location (address, city, state) to 4HELP (44357) for immediate help.

National Human Trafficking Hotline: Connects victims and survivors of sex and labor trafficking with services and supports to get help and stay safe.

https://humantraffickinghotline.org/

Call 1-888-373-7888. Stating or writing the number as 1-888-3737-888 makes it easier to remember.

(TTY: 711)
Text 233733

Health care

Many public assistance programs require frequent updates to paperwork for eligibility requirements. If a family moves often, they may miss the reminders to complete this paperwork and lose health insurance coverage. Some insurance companies require patients to have an annual physical examination by their listed primary care provider in order to maintain coverage. Pediatricians can help families maintain their insurance with reminders to complete preventive physical examination and update their information with the insurance company. It is important to know what policies and services are in place to help any patients who are experiencing a lapse in insurance. Many insurance companies will help provide transportation to appointments or provide gas reimbursement. These services can help families attend appointments and reduce out-of-pocket costs. Shelters and drop-in centers may have a medical provider visit. Some shelters have a clinic on site. These resources can provide continuity of care when a patient is not able to attend an appointment in the office. School-based health clinics, mobile clinics, and vans can also ease the burden of traveling to an office for an appointment.

The National Health Care for Homeless Council has several resources, including clinical guides, Webinars, online courses, and live training events (https://www.nhchc.org/) to improve health care delivery and skills for providers working with patients who are experiencing homelessness.

Education

Thorough documentation of medical needs and immunizations in a resource that can travel with the patient can help avoid duplication of testing and gaps in services. Many families and youth are not aware that every state has a coordinator to help children and youth experiencing homelessness. Updated lists of State Coordinators and additional resources are available from the National Center for Homeless Education (https://nche.ed.gov/data/). Communities in Schools (https://www.communitiesinschools.org/) can help children and youth access resources and stay in school.

National Association for the Education of Homeless Children and Youth:

A national membership association dedicated to ensuring educational equity and excellence for children and youth experiencing homelessness. They include a fact sheet for school staff, teachers, principals, and other administrators: http://www2.ed.gov/policy/elsec/leg/essa/160315ehcyfactsheet072716.pdf.

https://naehcy.org/mission/
E-mail: info@naehcy.org
Phone: 866-862-2562
Fax: 612-430-6995

National Center for Homeless Education: Provides data, resources, and connection to the state health coordinator.

Phone: 1-800-308-2145
E-mail: homeless@serve.org
Find state coordinator at: http://www.serve.org/nche/states/state_resourcers.php

Legal

Despite protections in the law, many people do not receive services unless they have legal help. Health care providers can help with the documentation of health conditions and the need for a healthy environment, for example, documenting that a patient has asthma and cannot be exposed to smoke, mold, or rodents; or the need for a patient with diabetes to have electricity to keep insulin cold. The Legal Services Corporation has a link on its Web site to help find legal aid: https://www.lsc.gov/.

Advocacy

Policies matter. Legislative acts like the McKinney-Vento Act, Every Student Succeeds Act, and the Runaway and Homeless Youth Act help in the definition of and development of services for runaway and homeless youth, but they cannot be fully effective without adequate funding and continued support from elected officials.[55]

The following actions can help with improving health for children and adolescents who are experiencing homelessness or who are at risk of becoming homeless:

- Supporting and following the provisions of the UN Conventions on the Rights of the Child[24,56]
- Universal health coverage[1–3,24,56]
- Increased awareness of health issues common among those experiencing homelessness or housing instability[2,22]
- Assistance with connecting at-risk families and youth with resources to prevent homelessness or to exit homelessness[2,24]
- Partnering with community agencies[2,24,56]
- Increased affordable housing[1–3,57]
- Protection and expansion of funding for programs to support those families at risk of homelessness, such as WIC, SNAP, TANF, and so forth.[2,24,58]
- Increase in dentists trained to care for pediatric patients[31]
- Additional research into interventions that have helped prevent homelessness or help children, adolescents, and families exit homelessness[24]

MODELS FOR PREVENTION

"Housing-first" models have been successful at improving health outcomes for children, families, and unaccompanied people experiencing homelessness. Some medical facilities are using their resources to provide a stable environment for patients in an effort to reduce readmissions.[57] These interventions can improve health outcomes for the patients and financial outcomes for institutions.[57]

Increased access to low-income housing prevents homelessness.[57] For those in shelter, access to health care, including age-appropriate dental and ophthalmologic services, and educational resources can improve outcomes for children and adolescents.[2,24,27,30–33]

Policies of the shelters also impact health care access. In Massachusetts, there was a more than 13-fold increase in the number of children presenting to the emergency department after a policy change requiring documentation of homelessness in order to access shelter.[59] Regular meetings among the various stakeholders, including those being served by programs, can help to avoid duplication of services and meet the changing needs of the communities.[24]

By treating every visit as an opportunity to meet acute and preventive health care needs, pediatricians can improve immunizations rates, decrease morbidity, and provide links to community services.[22] The lifecycle model shows that youth are more likely to exit the streets during times of crisis or disequilibrium. This time is also when they are likely to seek medical care.[10]

Mentorship programs for those who have survived CSE show some promise in decreasing health risks and continued exploitation.[21] Colleagues in family medicine, obstetrics and gynecology, and neonatology can help identify at-risk families before they are referred to pediatric care.

ROLE OF TECHNOLOGY IN CAUSING OR MANAGING THE ISSUE

Many homeless youth and families will keep a cell phone or access the Internet at libraries, schools, coffee shops, or public spaces. Using patient portals of the electronic medical records may be a feasible way of staying in contact because phone numbers and addresses may change often. They can also help the patient have a record of past treatment to share with new providers when they move. Youth experiencing homelessness report continued access to the Internet and smart phones, but use is significantly less frequent than housed youth.[60] Having "charging stations" in clinic can help many patients and their families, including those who are stably housed.

SUMMARY

Pediatricians are caring for a large and growing segment of the homeless population. Many patients and their families may not disclose their status because of concerns about stigma or lack of awareness of their situation. Pediatric providers can use their unique relationship with patients and their families to help them connect to resources to avoid or exit homelessness. Pediatricians must continue the strong tradition of advocacy to encourage legislation to prevent and reduce homelessness.

DISCLOSURE

The authors have nothing to disclose.

REFERENCES

1. National Healthcare for the Homeless Council. Medicare for all and the HCH community. 2019. Available at: https://www.nhchc.org/wp-content/uploads/2019/05/medicare-for-all-and-the-hch-community.pdf. Accessed July 27, 2019.
2. Council on Community Pediatrics. Providing care for children and adolescents facing homelessness and housing insecurity. Pediatrics 2013;131(6):1206–10.
3. National Healthcare for the Homeless Council. Mainstreaming health care for homeless people. 2005. Available at: https://nhchc.org/wp-content/uploads/2019/08/Mainstreaming-Health-Care-for-Homeless-People.pdf. Accessed October 22, 2019.
4. National Coalition for the Homeless. NCH fact sheet #18. McKinney-Vento Act. Published by the National Coalition for the Homeless. 2006. Available at: http://nationalhomeless.org/publications/facts/McKinney.pdf. Accessed July 27, 2019.
5. Youth.gov. "Youth topics, runaway and homeless youth, federal definitions". Available at: https://youth.gov/youth-topics/runaway-and-homeless-youth/federal-definitions#_ftn. Accessed July 27, 2019.
6. 34 USC Crime Control And Law Enforcement Subtitle I Comprehensive Acts. Chapter 111 juvenile justice and delinquency prevention, subchapter iii: runaway

and homeless youth. §11279. Definitions (3). Available at: https://uscode.house.gov/view.xhtml?path=/prelim@title34/subtitle1/chapter111/subchapter3&edition=prelim#11279_1. Accessed July 27, 2019.

7. Department Of Housing And Urban Development. Homeless emergency assistance and rapid transition to housing: emergency solutions grants program and consolidated plan conforming amendments. Federal Register 2011; 76(233):75954–94.

8. United States Interagency Council on Homelessness. Homelessness in America: focus on families with children. Available at: https://www.usich.gov/tools-for-action/homelessness-in-america-focus-on-families-with-children. Accessed July 27, 2019.

9. Auerswald CL, Eyre SL. Youth homelessness in San Francisco: a life cycle approach. Social Sci Med 2002;54(10):1497–512.

10. Carlson JL, Sugano E, Millstein SG, et al. Service utilization and the life cycle of youth homelessness. J Adolesc Health 2006;38(5):624–7.

11. National Coalition for the Homeless. Current state of homelessness 2018. Available at: http://nationalhomeless.org/wp-content/uploads/2018/04/State-of-things-2018-for-web.pdf. Accessed July 27, 2019.

12. Auerswald CL, Adams S. Counting all homeless youth today so we may no longer need to tomorrow. J Adolesc Health 2018;62(1):1–2.

13. Narendorf SC, Santa Maria DM, Ha Y, et al. Counting and surveying homeless youth: recommendations from YouthCount 2.0!, a community-academic partnership. J Community Health 2016;41(6):1234–41.

14. The US Department of Housing and Urban Development Office of Community Planning Development. The 2018 Annual Homeless Assessment Report (AHAR) to Congress. Part 1: Point in Time Estimates of Homelessness. Dec 2018. Available at: https://files.hudexchange.info/resources/documents/2018-AHAR-Part-1.pdf.

15. Brown SR, Shinn M, Khadduri J. Homeless families research brief: Well-being of young children after experiencing homelessness. 2017. Available at: https://www.acf.hhs.gov/sites/default/files/opre/opre_homefam_brief3_hhs_children_02_24_2017_b508.pdf. Accessed February 4, 2020.

16. Morton MH, Dworsky A, Matjasko JL, et al. Prevalence and correlates of youth homelessness in the United States. J Adolesc Health 2018;62(1):14–21.

17. National Center for Homeless Education. National overview. Available at: http://profiles.nche.seiservices.com/ConsolidatedStateProfile.aspx. Accessed July 28, 2019.

18. U.S. Department of Health and Human Services, Office of the Assistant Secretary of Planning and Evaluation (2017). Factors associated with prolonged youth homelessness. Available at: https://aspe.hhs.gov/pdf-report/factors-associatedprolonged-youth-homelessness. Accessed July, 28, 2019.

19. Rice E. The TAY triage tool: a tool to identify homeless transition age youth most in need of permanent supportive housing. 2013. Available at: http://www.csh.org/wp-content/uploads/2014/02/TAY_TriageTool_2014.pdf. Accessed July 28, 2019.

20. US Department of State. Trafficking in persons report June 2019. Available at: https://www.state.gov/reports/2019-trafficking-in-persons-report/. Accessed February 4, 2020.

21. Rothman EF, Preis SR, Bright K, et al. A longitudinal evaluation of a survivor-mentor program for child survivors of sex trafficking in the United States. Child Abuse Negl 2019;100:104083.

22. Karr C, Kline S. Homeless children: what every clinician should know. Pediatr Rev 2004;25(7):235–41.

23. Radcliff E, Crouch E, Strompolis M, et al. Homelessness in childhood and adverse childhood experiences (ACEs). Matern Child Health J 2019;23(6):811–20.

24. Society for Adolescent Health and Medicine. The healthcare needs and rights of youth experiencing homelessness. J Adolesc Health 2018;63(3):372–5.

25. Sandel M, Sheward R, Ettinger de Cuba S, et al. Timing and duration of pre- and postnatal homelessness and the health of young children. Pediatrics 2018;142(4) [pii:e20174254].

26. Sakai-Bizmark R, Chang RR, Mena LA, et al. Asthma hospitalizations among homeless children in New York State. Pediatrics 2019;144(2) [pii:e20182769].

27. Rodriguez J, Applebaum J, Stephenson-Hunter C, et al. Cooking, healthy eating, fitness and fun (CHEFFS): qualitative evaluation of a nutrition education program for children living at urban family homeless shelters. Am J Public Health 2013; 103(Suppl 2):S361–7.

28. Hartline-Grafton H. Understanding the connections: food insecurity and obesity. 2015. Available at: http://frac.org/pdf/frac_brief_understanding_the_connections. pdf. Accessed July 31, 2019.

29. de Grubb M, Levine RS, Zoorob RJ. Diet and obesity issues in the underserved. Prim Care 2017;44(1):127–40.

30. Chi D, Milgrom P. The oral health of homeless adolescents and young adults and determinants of oral health: preliminary findings. Spec Care Dentist 2008;28(6): 237–42.

31. Vargas CM, Ronzio CR. Disparities in early childhood caries. BMC Oral Health 2006;6:S3.

32. Barnes AJ, Lafavor TL, Cutuli JJ, et al. Health and self-regulation among school-age children experiencing family homelessness. Children (Basel) 2017;4(8) [pii:E70].

33. Smith NL, Smith TJ, DeSantis D, et al. Vision problems in homeless children. J Health Care Poor Underserved 2015;26(3):761–70.

34. Mackelprang JL, Qiu Q, Rivara FP. Predictors of emergency department visits and inpatient admissions among homeless and unstably housed adolescents and young adults. Med Care 2015;53(12):1010–7.

35. Holland DP, Alexander S, Onwubiko U, et al. Response to isoniazid-resistant tuberculosis in homeless shelters, Georgia, USA, 2015–2017. Emerg Infect Dis 2019;25(3):593–5.

36. Bonilla DL, Cole-Porse C, Kjemtrup A, et al. Risk factors for human lice and bartonellosis among the homeless, San Francisco, California, USA. Emerg Infect Dis 2014;20(10):1645–51.

37. Probert WS, Gonzalez C, Espinosa A, et al. Molecular genotyping of hepatitis A virus, California, USA, 2017–2018. Emerg Infect Dis 2019;25(8):1594–6.

38. Boonyaratanakornkit J, Ekici Seda, Magaret A, et al. Respiratory syncytial virus infection in homeless populations, Washington, USA. Emerg Infect Dis 2019; 25(7):1408–11.

39. Caccamo A, Kachur R, Williams SP. Narrative review: sexually transmitted diseases and homeless youth—what do we know about sexually transmitted disease prevalence and risk? Sex Transm Dis 2017;44(8):466–76.

40. Medlow S, Klineberg E, Steinbeck K. The health diagnoses of homeless adolescents: a systematic review of the literature. Ment Health J Adolesc 2014;37(5): 531–42.

41. Edinburgh L, Pape-Blabolil J, Harpin S, et al. Assessing exploitation experiences of girls and boys seen at a child advocacy center. Child Abuse Negl 2015;46: 47–59.

42. Thrane LE, Chen X. Impact of running away on girls' pregnancy. J Adolesc 2012; 35(2):443–9.
43. Thompson SJ, Bender KA, Lewis CM, et al. Runaway and pregnant: risk factors associated with pregnancy in a national sample of runaway/homeless female adolescents. J Adolesc Health 2008;43(2):125–32.
44. Crawford DM, Trotter EC, Hartshorn KJ, et al. Pregnancy and mental health of young homeless women. Am J Orthopsychiatry 2011;81(2):173–83.
45. Whitbeck LB, Johnson KD, Hoyt DR, et al. Mental disorder and comorbidity among runaway and homeless adolescents. J Adolesc Health 2004;35(2): 132–40.
46. Stewart AJ, Steiman M, Cauce AM, et al. Victimization and posttraumatic stress disorder among homeless adolescents. J Am Acad Child Adolesc Psychiatry 2004;43:325–31.
47. Barnes AJ, Gilbertson J, Chatterjee D. Emotional health among youth experiencing family homelessness. Pediatrics 2018;141(4) [pii:e20171767].
48. Ginzler JA, Garrett SB, Baer JS, et al. Measurement of negative consequences of substance use in street youth: an expanded use of the Rutgers Alcohol Problem Index. Addict Behav 2007;32:1519–25.
49. Barman-Adhikari A, Hsu HT, Brydon D, et al. Prevalence and correlates of nonmedical use of prescription drugs (NMUPD) among young adults experiencing homelessness in seven cities across the United States. Drug Alcohol Depend 2019;200:153–60.
50. Obradović J, Long JD, Cutuli JJ, et al. Academic achievement of homeless and highly mobile children in an urban school district: longitudinal evidence on risk, growth, and resilience. Dev Psychopathol 2009;21(2):493–518.
51. Sandel M, Sheward R, Ettinger de Cuba S, et al. Unstable housing and caregiver and child health in renter families. Pediatrics 2018;141(2).
52. Feldman BJ, Calogero CG, Elsayed KS, et al. Prevalence of homelessness in the emergency department setting. West J Emerg Med 2017;18(3):366–72.
53. Cohen E, Mackenzie RG, Yates GL. HEADSS, a psychosocial risk assessment instrument: implications for designing effective intervention programs for runaway youth. J Adolesc Health 1991;12(7):539–44.
54. Hornor G, Quinones SG, Bretl D, et al. Commercial sexual exploitation of children: an update for the forensic nurse. J Forensic Nurs 2019;15(2):93–102.
55. Dreyer BP. A shelter is not a home: the crisis of family homelessness in the United States. Pediatrics 2018;142(5) [pii: e20182695].
56. Scott BH, Elliott AS, Auerswald CL. A moral case for universal healthcare for runaway and homeless youth. Int J Hum Rights Healthc 2017;10(3):195–202.
57. Sandel M, Desmond M. Investing in housing for health improves both mission and margin. JAMA 2017;318(23):2291–2.
58. Richards R, Merrill RM, Baksh L, et al. Maternal health behaviors and infant health outcomes among homeless mothers: U.S. Special supplemental nutrition program for women, infants, and children (WIC) 2000-2007. Prev Med 2011;52(1): 87–94.
59. Stewart AM, Kanak MM, Gerald AM, et al. Pediatric emergency department visits for homelessness after shelter eligibility policy change. Pediatrics 2018;142(5) [pii: e20181224] (Increase in Peds ED visit after Policy change).
60. VonHoltz LAH, Frasso R, Golinkoff JM, et al. Internet and social media access among youth experiencing homelessness: mixed-methods study. J Med Internet Res 2018;20(5):e184.

Substance Use Disorders in Vulnerable Children

Andrew Spaedy, MD[a], Stacy Doumas, MD[a,b], Ramon Solhkhah, MD[a,b],*

KEYWORDS

- Substance use disorder • Vulnerable children • Comorbid psychiatric condition

KEY POINTS

- Substance use remains a major challenge in adolescent health.
- The coexisting use of these substances often creates hurdles for accurate diagnosis of other comorbid psychiatric conditions.
- It is of critical importance that health care providers be aware of both the isolated presentation of substance use disorder (SUC) as well as that with coexisting psychiatric illness.

INTRODUCTION

Adolescent substance use is a critically important topic, particularly to practicing pediatricians. Despite recent studies suggesting that substance use is decreasing among adolescents, their use is still high enough to remain of concern.[1,2] Adolescents with a substance use disorder show a high prevalence of psychiatric disorders as compared with age-matched peers that are not using substances.[3–9] Many of these individuals are also faced with nonsubstance use disorder comorbid psychiatric disorders. Meeting the needs of children and families via identifying and fully treating youth with substance use can be challenging, as these patients often present in ways that are unique compared with those of their adult counterparts. It is for this reason that an understanding of many of the most commonly used/abused substances by adolescents, along with common coexisting psychiatric conditions is relevant, particularly in vulnerable and at-risk children. This article reviews various commonly used substances, their diagnosis, epidemiology, treatment, and common coexisting psychiatric conditions in vulnerable youth, along with the effect of parental substance use on adolescents.

[a] Department of Psychiatry, Jersey Shore University Medical Center, 1945 State Route 33, Rosa 105 D, Neptune, NJ 07753, USA; [b] Department of Psychiatry & Behavioral Health, Hackensack Meridian School of Medicine at Seton Hall University, 340 Kingsland Street, Nutley, NJ 07710, USA
* Corresponding author.
E-mail address: ramon.solhkhah@hackensackmeridian.org

Pediatr Clin N Am 67 (2020) 373–385
https://doi.org/10.1016/j.pcl.2019.11.002
0031-3955/20/© 2019 Elsevier Inc. All rights reserved.

SUBSTANCES AND THEIR TREATMENT
Alcohol

Alcohol is likely the greatest concern when it comes to adolescent substance use. Alcohol use in the adult population accounts for a significant portion of emergency room visits in the United States, and is growing; the period 2006 to 2014 saw a nearly 50% increase in emergency room visits among US adults.[1] Although it is true that alcohol-related visits to the emergency department in the adolescent population are not as high, it remains an important topic that clinicians who work with adolescents must be familiar with. As per the 2018 *Monitoring the Future* study, at the time adolescents reach the end of high school nearly 60% have drank alcohol (more than just a "few sips"), and nearly 1 in 4 had consumed alcohol by the eighth grade.[2]

There are well-researched screening tools that clinicians may find useful when evaluating adolescents for alcohol use disorder. The first is the *CRAFFT* questionnaire, which is a 6-question assessment composed of the following questions—C: Have you ever ridden in a *car* driven by someone (including yourself) who was "high" or using alcohol or drugs? R: Do you use alcohol or drugs to *relax*, change your mood, feel better about yourself, or fit in? A: Do you ever use alcohol or drugs while you are by yourself, *alone*? F: Has any *friend, family* member, or other person ever thought you had a problem with alcohol or drugs? F: Do you ever *forget* (or regret) things you did while using? T: Have you ever gotten into *trouble* while using alcohol or drugs, or done something you would not normally do (break the law, rules, or curfew; engage in risky behavior to you or others)?[10] The CRAFFT screening tool has been shown to be able to identify 86% of individuals with alcohol use disorders.[11,12]

The PESQ (Personal Experience Screening Questionnaire) is another tool that may be used. Unlike the CRAFFT, the PESQ is not in the public domain; however, what it carries in expense it may make up for in its more thorough questioning. It covers drug use history, psychosocial problems, as well as the ability to unveil distortion tendencies, such as the participant faking good or bad. When empirically derived cutoffs were utilized, the PESQ was found to correctly identify 87% of cases of alcohol use disorders.[12]

In the emergency department, laboratory tests that may aid in the diagnosis include: blood alcohol concentration, mean corpuscular volume to look for macrocytosis, carbohydrate-deficient transferrin, as well as aspartate aminotransferase and alanine aminotransferase.[13] Generally, individuals with mild intoxication will only require observation, serial physical/mental status examinations, and supportive care. More severe intoxication may require aggressive supportive care, respiratory and blood pressure monitoring. Although significantly less likely in adolescents than the adult population, individuals with heavy chronic use, may develop delirium tremens. This potentially life-threatening condition, while rare, when present requires benzodiazepines, thiamine, and intravenous (IV) fluids.[14]

Vaping and Other Tobacco Products

Although cigarettes and, to a lesser extent, chewing tobacco, have historically been the major source of tobacco products consumed by adolescents, vaporized e-cigarettes, or vaping, have, in recent years, made a tremendous mark of their own. Vaping involves using a battery-powered device to heat a plant or chemical liquid material resulting in an aerosol. This aerosol often contains nicotine in addition to a flavoring medium, which may come in a myriad of different flavors including, but not limited to: bubblegum, fruit, and chocolate—all of which cater to a younger population over their traditional cigarette counterpart.

As previously stated, the adoption of vaping by adolescents in recent years has been significant. In fact, 1 long-term study found it to have the greatest increase of year over year use for any substance, out of the last 44 years that the data have been tracked.[2] Usage rates of nicotine vaping reached 30% in individuals in the 12th grade. This is especially concerning given that vaping seems to predict experimentation in the future with cigarettes.[15,16] It is worrisome that this trend may signal a slowing or even reversal in the trend that has been observed over the last 2 decades of decreasing cigarette smoking among adolescents. Some possible reasons for their popularity include that adolescents view them as having the lowest perceived risk of all drugs, a declining of perceived risk with increasing age, as well as a comparatively low disapproval of regular e-cigarette use compared with that of other substances.[2]

Although the number of individuals who vape nicotine is increasing, there are still a significant population of adolescents who are consuming both smoked and smokeless tobacco. Fortunately, there has been considerable decreases over the last 2 decades in smoking prevalence in youth. By 2018, the 30-day prevalence level had decreased by 75% to 90% for adolescents between grades 8 to 12. As cigarette smoking is the leading cause of preventable disease and mortality in the United States, it is critical to continue combating it at the forefront of public health.[2]

Issues of nicotine withdrawal or intoxication generally do not require emergency department care. One exception to this is accidental ingestion—usually by young children. This results in symptoms, such as mucosal irritation, nausea, headache, and diaphoresis, as well as both tachycardia and bradyarrhythmias. Care is generally supportive; however, telemetry may be beneficial to monitor for the aforementioned arrhythmias.[17]

3,4-Methylenedioxymethamphetamine

Club drugs include such substances as 3,4-methylenedioxymethamphetamine (MDMA), ketamine, and gamma hydroxybutyrate. They originally received their name from their popular use in clubs and rave parties. MDMA, also known as "ecstasy," "Molly," and a host of other street names, is a stimulant-like mild hallucinogen. It is chemically similar to the stimulant amphetamine and the hallucinogen mescaline. It is generally taken orally in tablet or capsule form with an onset of action between 30 and 60 minutes and an active effect between 3 and 6 hours.[18] Intoxication consists of 3 stages: disorientation, "tingling and spasmodic jerking," and finally increased sociability, mental clarity, a feeling of well-being and closeness to others. Post-use effects include a period of 24 to 48 hours of confusion, depression, insomnia, anxiety, and paranoia.[19,20] Typical adverse reactions from MDMA are generally minor and include "agitation, nausea, bruxism, ataxia, diaphoresis, blurry vision, tachycardia, and hypertension."[21] These reactions are generally self-limited and resolve within hours with supportive care. More severe side effects, while uncommon, such as hypertensive emergency, arrhythmias, hyperthermia, hyponatremia, hepatotoxicity, and serotonin syndrome may also occur in a subset of patients and require specialized treatment.[22–25]

Marijuana

Marijuana is derived from the *Cannabis sativa* plant. Its major psychoactive component is delta-9-tetrahydrocannabinol (THC) along with at least 60 other cannabinoids.[26,27] Marijuana may be smoked or orally ingested. Psychoactive effects of smoked marijuana occur rapidly with onset at 15 to 30 minutes lasting up to 4 hours.

Typically, doses of 2 to 3 mg of THC are sufficient to produce drug effects in drug-naive individuals. Ingested marijuana has a relatively slower onset ranging between 30 minutes and 3 hours; its active effect may last up to 12 hours with an effective dose between 5 and 20 mg of THC in naive users.[26,27] The physiologic signs of intoxication with cannabis may include the following: conjunctival injection, dry mouth, increased appetite, tachycardia, hypertension, tachypnea, slurred speech, nystagmus, and ataxia.[26,28]

The use of marijuana is extremely prevalent among US adolescents. According to the Monitoring the Future study, it is the single most used illicit drug since the study began 44 years ago.[2] At present, 1 in 17 high school seniors smoke marijuana daily—representing a sharp increase in recent years. This increased use is likely due in part to a concomitant decrease in perceived risk coupled (partially driven by the legalized/medicinal marijuana movement) with decreased personal disapproval of use among adolescents, and increased accessibility of marijuana-based vaping products.

Treatment of marijuana intoxication is rarely indicated. However, there are medications that have been trialed as adjuncts to psychosocial treatments, the most promising of which include N-acetylcysteine, valproate, and gabapentin.[29]

Cocaine

Cocaine, possibly the most potent stimulant of natural origin, is an extract from the coca plant (*Erythroxylum coca*). It exerts its effects via blockade of the reuptake of several biogenic amines (ie, dopamine, norepinephrine, and epinephrine), sodium channel blockade (contributing to its analgesic effect), and exciting amino acid (ie, glutamate and aspartate) stimulation. Clinical manifestations of intoxication include the following: dose-dependent increases in blood pressure and heart rate, euphoria, arousal, improved performance on tasks, alertness, and a sense of self-confidence. Discontinuation may result in a state of dysphoria and depressive symptoms.

Not infrequently, cocaine intoxication may result in psychotic symptoms. This may present as tactile hallucinations—such as bugs crawling on the skin—known as formication. Paranoia is also possible. Psychotic symptoms usually self-resolve within 48 to 72 hours of cocaine cessation. Cocaine has also been associated with a myriad of other adverse effects affecting the cardiovascular (myocardial infarction), central nervous (seizures, coma, headache, intracranial hemorrhage, and focal neurologic symptoms), pulmonary (pulmonary infarction and reversible airway disease), gastrointestinal (ulcer perforation), and renal (renal infarction) systems.[29–32]

Generally speaking, the management for cocaine intoxication is supportive. Certain medications, especially benzodiazepines, may be useful for the symptomatic treatment of agitation, such as diazepam or lorazepam. Occasionally the use of antipsychotic may be warranted. Seizures should be treated with antiepileptic drugs.

Among adolescents, cocaine use has been declining since 1999. Currently use is between 0.8% and 2.3% for individuals between grades 8 and 12.[2]

Opioids

Opiates are an extract from the poppy plant (*Papaver somniferum*). They belong to the larger class of drugs, opioids, which include both the synthetic and semi-synthetic drugs. Opioid receptors are present in both the central and peripheral nervous system.

They are tied to a variety of neurotransmitters, resulting in a diverse clinical picture of analgesia, euphoria, and anxiolysis.

Opioid overdose has been at the forefront of attention in the United States in recent years due to record high levels of overdose. In fact in 2017, 47,000 Americans died as a result of opioid overdose.[33] Overdose results in a potentially lethal clinical picture of respiratory depression, decreased mental status and bowel sounds, and miotic pupils. Almost immediate reversal can be achieved via administration of an opiate antagonist, naloxone.[34] Unlike overdose, withdrawal from opioids is generally safe, albeit uncomfortable. Clinical symptoms of withdrawal include dysphoria, restlessness, rhinorrhea, lacrimation, myalgias, arthralgias, nausea, emesis, abdominal cramping, and diarrhea.[35] Both buprenorphine and methadone have been used for the treatment of opioid dependence in the adolescent population.[36] Clonidine, an alpha-2-agonist, has also been found to be useful for the autonomic signs during the withdrawal period.[37]

Opioids are unquestionably a major public health problem. In the adolescent population, change for the better seems to be occurring. Since 2009, both heroin and other narcotic drug use has been at an all-time low in individuals in grades 8 to 12. Although usage rates are still fairly high in this age group, usage rates have decreased from 9.2% to 3.4% over the last 10 years.[2]

CO-OCCURRING PSYCHIATRIC DISORDERS IN ADOLESCENTS
Depressive Disorders

A significant amount has been written about the relationship between depression and substance use.[38–48] In adolescents[38,40,41,49] and adults[42–44] there are 2 distinct groups of patients: those with a substance-induced mood disorder and those with a primary depressive disorder. Depression is characterized by sadness as well as a loss of interest or pleasure. It is important to note that adolescents may report or exhibit irritability instead of sadness. In addition you may see guilt, hopelessness, sleep disturbances, issues with appetite, inability to concentrate, and poor energy, as well as thoughts of suicide and death. Depressed adolescents may benefit from certain cognitive interventions for depression.[50,51]

Stressful childhood experiences, such as trauma and depressive symptoms, have been associated with the start of drug use. Fishbein and colleagues[52] examined the lifetime traumatic stressors and their intensity of the onset of drug use and the subsequent risk of development of depressive symptoms. They found that drug use initiation during early adolescence (age 14–16 years) may not be tied to immediate proximal disturbances in risk factors, such as trauma and depressive symptoms. Instead, the effects of trauma on depression, in the sample examined, seem to be established earlier in childhood (before age 14 years). These effects then persist into middle adolescence where the risk for drug use is then heightened.

In 1 study, 126 adolescents with a DSM IV diagnosis for major depressive disorder, substance use disorder (SUD), and conduct disorder were studied to examine the efficacy of fluoxetine compared with placebo. Cognitive behavioral therapy was administered in both groups for their SUD during the 16 weeks. Post-trial, rates of depression were high in both groups—64% for the placebo group versus 75% for fluoxetine—however, rates of abstinence were low. Ultimately it was concluded that remission of depression was a stronger predictor of change in drug use than medication treatment. Symptoms of depression may remit via individual outpatient cognitive behavioral therapy (CBT) for SUD without pharmacotherapy; however, if symptoms do not improve in the first month of treatment, fluoxetine is critical because ongoing depression may prevent reaching abstinence.[53–55]

Bipolar Disorder

The diagnosis of bipolar disorder can be especially challenging to make in patients who have not reached adulthood and it is made even more difficult concert with the use of drugs and alcohol. Although certain symptoms, such as changes in sleeping patterns and mood swings may include symptoms of bipolar disorder, they are also characteristic of both substance use and normal adolescence. With that said, a diagnosis of bipolar disorder should be considered in youth who use substances, especially those who are binge users. Bipolar disorder often begins in late adolescence,[56–58] with symptomatology of mania and depression. Mania is characterized by a persistently elevated, expansive or irritable mood of at least 1 week, a decreased need for sleep, speech that is pressured, racing thoughts, increased purposeful activity, and excessive involvement in pleasurable activities, such as sex and substance use.

Wilens and colleagues, found that there was an increased risk for SUD in adolescents with bipolar disorder. They reported an 8.8-fold increase in SUD with adolescent onset bipolar disorder compared with childhood onset bipolar disorder. Children who were diagnosed and treated appropriately at a younger age had a lower overall risk for SUD.[58] Goldstein and Bukstein[59] also examined the burden of SUD in youth with bipolar disorder. According to their report, youth onset bipolar disorder confers an even greater risk of SUD when compared with adult onset bipolar disorder.

Pharmacotherapy should be initiated once a diagnosis of bipolar disorder is established. Lithium, valproic acid, carbamazepine, and other anticonvulsants are typically effective. Atypical antipsychotics, such as olanzapine and risperidone are also options.[58,60,61] Of note, in a study by Geller, [62–64] lithium was able to not only control the symptoms of mania, but also to decrease the use of alcohol.

Anxiety Disorders

Anxiety disorders are among the most often coexisting psychiatric disorders in adolescents and adults with SUD. The following conditions may all be considered to be under the umbrella of anxiety disorders discussed in this section: generalized anxiety disorder, obsessive-compulsive disorder, panic disorder, social phobia, and posttraumatic stress disorder. Unfortunately, anxiety disorders are frequently not detected, especially when in the presence of depression or SUD.[56,65]

Frojd and colleagues[66] examined the relationship of anxiety to alcohol and other substance use, along with whether anxiety or other social phobia symptoms affect the continuity of frequent alcohol use, drunkenness, and cannabis use. They determined that anxiety preceded substance use while no reciprocal associations were observed. This study suggests that general anxiety in middle adolescents may place a youth at risk for concurrent and subsequent substance use.

Many children with social phobia may not be recognized early due to a lack of classroom behavioral issues. However, aggressive children are frequently referred for psychiatric evaluation. In these patients it is critical to carefully evaluate the youngster for anxiety disorders, such as social phobia. In 1 study, it was found that the combination of aggressiveness and shyness in male adolescents was a superior predictor of future cocaine use than that of a history of aggressiveness alone.[67]

There also seems to be gender differences in the co-occurrence of type of anxiety disorder as well as the type of substance used in adolescents. A study by Wu and colleagues[68] examined this phenomena in a study of 781 adolescents aged between 13 and 17 years. They found that social phobia was strongly associated with cigarette smoking among boys only, whereas girls actually had a negative association with drug use. Among the other SUDs, the correlation with substance use tended to be stronger with girls. This draws attention to the need for improved clinical recognition of anxiety disorder as well as the need to improve treatment access to the youth struggling with these conditions.

Posttraumatic Stress Disorder

Posttraumatic stress disorder (PTSD) deserves special attention in the adolescent population, as clinical reports have found a high incidence of trauma and PTSD symptoms among these individuals.[65,69,70] Symptoms, such as memories of a past traumatic event, may be intensified during periods of abstinence, resulting in adolescents using substances as a means to escape.

Adolescents exposed to multiple forms of psychological trauma may be at high risk for both behavioral and psychiatric disorders. In a recent study by Ford and colleagues,[71] 6 mutually exclusive trauma profiles were identified in adolescents. Four of these classes were found to have a high likelihood of poly-victimization: including victims of abuse (8%), victims of physical assault (9%), and victims of community violence (15.5%). Individuals of poly-victimization were more likely than youth traumatized by witnessing violence or exposure to disaster/accident trauma to have psychiatric diagnosis and (independent of psychiatric diagnoses or demographics) to be involved in delinquency than delinquent peers. Poly-victimization is common in adolescents, and it places these youth at a higher risk for psychiatric disease and delinquency.

Trauma and its related symptoms should be inquired about by health care professionals to ensure that adequate treatment can be provided to substance using adolescents. Referrals to groups that promote self-care and a first-things-first attitude could be the best approach. In addition, integrated PTSD and SUD focused cognitive behavioral therapy, as well as family treatment for adolescents with comorbid abuse-related PTSD and SUD, could optimize the outcome for these patients.[72]

PARENTAL SUBSTANCE USE AND CHILD WELFARE

Medical professionals caring for adolescents need to be aware of the significant relationship between parental substance use and child maltreatment. In 1 study, it was found that children whose caregivers were abusing substances were 2.7 times more likely to be abused and 4.2 times more likely to be neglected.[33,73,74] In another study, in 43% of juvenile court cases of serious child abuse or neglect, at least 1 parent had a documented substance use issue.[75] Parents who are acutely intoxicated or withdrawing do not respond appropriately to the cues that their children give, resulting in basic needs going unmet. In addition, there are many drugs of abuse that can cause adult caregivers to become angry, paranoid, and violent; this brews a situation in which the child may be prone to injury from their parent.[76] If this was not enough, children raised in these settings are at increased risk for abusing substances as they grow older.[77]

Homes in which illicit drugs or alcohol are being abused have many environmental risks to the children living there. These places may contain hazards, such as unsanitary living conditions, domestic violence, pornography, and criminal activity.[78] They may be exposed to drugs directly via accidental ingestion or second-hand smoke.[79–81] Unsafe materials, such as needles—if the caregiver is an IV drug user— may be present and can cause injury.

Unfortunately caregivers intentionally giving their children drugs is also an issue. There are at least 3 cases where mothers administered methadone to their children to sedate them. In all cases the children died as a result of the ingestion, resulting in all 3 subsequent court cases being ruled as homicides.[82,83] There have also been reports of forced ingestion of illicit substance and alcohol for the entertainment of the caregiver. One study found that 11% of babysitters blew smoke in the faces of the children that they were supervising.[84]

A detailed social history is of paramount importance for practitioners caring for children to accurately identify children who may be in these troubling living situations. It is recommended that a nonjudgmental inquiry be made as to which drugs are being used in the home, and to what extent. This information may be critical for the diagnosis for the adolescent patient, as well as help to identify areas that support may be needed for the whole family.

Because of the serious and recurring nature of drug addiction, ensuring the safety of the children in households with addicted parents is critical. Reporting laws require that medical providers report cases of confirmed or suspected child neglect or abuse. Reporting can often help to facilitate a home safety evaluation in addition to a review of previous or potential welfare concerns of the family. In addition, it may help to smooth the path of getting the addicted caregiver into treatment and recovery programs.

SUMMARY

Substance use remains a major challenge in adolescent health. The coexisting use of these substances often creates hurdles for accurate diagnosis of other comorbid psychiatric conditions. It is of critical importance that health care providers be aware of both the isolated presentation of SUD as well as that with coexisting psychiatric illness. In some cases psycho-pharmacotherapy may be of benefit. Given the continued discovery of new treatment options, treatment providers must stay up to date.[61] Youth should also be encouraged to take part in appropriate therapy, via CBT, Al-a-teen, Alcoholics Anonymous, Narcotics Anonymous.[85–88] Finally, special care must be taken to identify and properly assist youth in homes with substance abusing parents. These patients, if not properly assisted, are at risk for a myriad of troubling situations.

REFERENCES

1. NIH study shows steep increase in rate of alcohol-related ER visits. Available at: https://www.niaaa.nih.gov/news-events/news-releases/nih-study-shows-steep-increase-rate-alcohol-related-er-visits. Accessed July 27, 2019.
2. Johnston LD, O'Malley PM, Miech RA, et al. Monitoring the future national survey results on drug use, 1975–2018: overview, key findings on adolescent drug use. Ann Arbor (MI): Institute for Social Research, The University of Michigan; 2019.
3. Hovens JG, Cantwell DP, Kiriakos R. Psychiatric comorbidity in hospitalized adolescent substance abusers. J Am Acad Child Adolesc Psychiatry 1994; 33(4):476–83.
4. Brook JS, Whiteman M, Cohen P, et al. Longitudinally predicting late adolescent and young adult drug use: childhood and adolescent precursors. J Am Acad Child Adolesc Psychiatry 1995;34:1230–8.
5. Christie KA, Burke JD, Regier DA, et al. Epidemiologic evidence for early onset of mental disorders and higher risk of drug abuse in young adults. Am J Psychiatry 1988;145:971–5.
6. DeMilio L. Psychiatric syndromes in adolescent substance abusers. Am J Psychiatry 1989;146:1212–4.

7. Kaminer Y. The magnitude of concurrent psychiatric disorders in hospitalized substance abusing adolescents. J Abnorm Child Psychol 1991;25:122–32.
8. Kandel DB, Johnson JG, Bird H, et al. Psychiatric disorders associated with substance use among children and adolescents: findings from the methods for the epidemiology of child and adolescent mental disorders (MECA) study. J Abnorm Child Psychol 1997;25:122–32.
9. Kellam SG, Ensminger ME, Simon MB. Mental health in first grade and teenage drug, alcohol, and cigarette use. Drug Alcohol Depend 1980;5:273–304.
10. Winters KC, Kaminer Y. Screening and assessing adolescent substance use disorders in clinical populations. J Am Acad Child Adolesc Psychiatry 2008;47(7): 740–4.
11. Knight JR, Sherritt L, Shrier LA, et al. Validity of the CRAFFT substance abuse screening test among adolescent clinic patients. Arch Pediatr Adolesc Med 2002;156(6):607–14.
12. Knight JR, Sherritt L, Harris SK, et al. Validity of brief alcohol screening tests among adolescents: a comparison of the AUDIT, POSIT, CAGE, and CRAFFT. Alcohol Clin Exp Res 2003;27(1):67–73.
13. Jastrzębska I, Zwolak A, Szczyrek M, et al. Biomarkers of alcohol misuse: recent advances and future prospects. Prz Gastroenterol 2016;11(2):78–89.
14. Bird RD, Makela EH. Alcohol withdrawal: what is the benzodiazepine of choice? Ann Pharmacother 1994;28(1):67–71.
15. Miech RA, Patrick ME, O'Malley PM, et al. Ecigarette use as a predictor of cigarette smoking: Results from a 1-year follow-up of a national sample of 12th grade students. Tob Control 2017;26(e2):e106–11.
16. Soneji S, Barrington-Trimis JL, Wills TA, et al. Association between initial use of ecigarettes and subsequent cigarette smoking among adolescents and young adults: a systematic review and meta-analysis. JAMA Pediatr 2017;171(8): 788–97.
17. Smolinske SC, Spoerke DG, Spiller SK, et al. Cigarette and nicotine chewing gum toxicity in children. Hum Toxicol 1988;7(1):27–31.
18. DA J. "Designer drugs"—a current perspective. PubMed, NCBI. [online] Ncbi.nlm.-nih.gov. 2019. Available at: https://www.ncbi.nlm.nih.gov/pubmed/2096172. Accessed July 27, 2019.
19. Parrott A, Lasky J. Ecstasy (MDMA) effects upon mood and cognition: before, during and after a Saturday night dance. Psychopharmacology 1998;139:261.
20. Cami J, Farré M, Mas M, et al. Human pharmacology of 3,4-methylenedioxymethamphetamine ("ecstasy"): psychomotor performance and subjective effects. J Clin Psychopharmacol 2019;20(4):455–66.
21. Thompson JP. Acute effects of drugs of abuse. Clin Med (Lond) 2003;3(2):123–6.
22. Lai T-I, Hwang J-J, Fang C-C, et al. Methylene 3,4-dioxymethamphetamine-induced acute myocardial infarction. Ann Emerg Med 2003;42(6):759–62.
23. Mas M, Farre M, de la Torre R, et al. Cardiovascular and neuroendocrine effects and pharmacokinetics of 3, 4-methylenedioxymethamphetamine in humans. J Pharmacol Exp Ther 1999;290(1):136–45.
24. Caballero F, Lopez-Navidad A, Cotorruelo J, et al. Ecstasy-induced brain death and acute hepatocellular failure: multiorgan donor and liver transplantation. Transplantation 2002;74(4):532–7.
25. Callaway CW, Clark RF. Hyperthermia in psychostimulant overdose. Ann Emerg Med 1994;24(1):68–76.
26. Grotenhermen F. Pharmacokinetics and pharmacodynamics of cannabinoids. Clin Pharmacokinet 2003;42(4):327–60.

27. Huestis MA. Human cannabinoid pharmacokinetics. Chem Biodivers 2007;4(8): 1770–804.
28. Adams IB, Martin BR. Cannabis: pharmacology and toxicology in animals and humans. Addiction 1996;91(11):1585–614.
29. Sherman BJ, McRae-Clark AL. Treatment of cannabis use disorder: current science and future outlook. Pharmacotherapy 2016;36(5):511–35.
30. Lange RA, Cigarroa RG, Yancy CWJ, et al. Cocaine-induced coronary-artery vasoconstriction. N Engl J Med 1989;321(23):1557–62.
31. Hoffman RS. Cocaine. In: Goldfrank LR, Flomenbaum NE, Hoffman RS, et al, editors. Goldfrank's toxicologic emergencies. 8th edition. New York: McGraw-Hill Medical Publishing Division; 2006. p. 1133.
32. Ettinger NA, Albin RJ. A review of the respiratory effects of smoking cocaine. Am J Med 1989;87(6):664–8.
33. White WL, Illinois Department of Children and Family Services, Illinois Department of Alcoholism and Substance Abuse. SAFE 95: a status report on Project Safe, an innovative project designed to break the cycle of maternal substance abuse and child neglect/abuse. Springfield (IL): Illinois Department of Children and Family Services; 1995.
34. Mills CA, Flacke JW, Flacke WE, et al. Narcotic reversal in hypercapnic dogs: comparison of naloxone and nalbuphine. Can J Anaesth 1990;37(2):238–44.
35. Stolbach A, Hoffman RS. Opioid withdrawal in the emergency setting. Waltham (MA): UpToDate Inc; 2019. Available at: https://www.uptodate.com/contents/opioid-withdrawal-in-the-emergency-setting. Accessed on July 20, 2019.
36. Gutwinski S, Bald LK, Gallinat J, et al. Why do patients stay in opioid maintenance treatment? Subst Use Misuse 2014;49(6):694–9.
37. Jasinski DR, Johnson RE, Kocher TR. Clonidine in morphine withdrawal: differential effects on signs and symptoms. Arch Gen Psychiatry 1985;42(11):1063–6.
38. Bukstein O, Glancy LJ, Kaminer Y. Patterns of affective comorbidity in a clinical population of dually diagnosed adolescent substance abusers. J Am Acad Child Adolesc Psychiatry 1992;31(6):1041–5.
39. Wilcox JA, Yates WR. Gender and psychiatric comorbidity in substance-abusing individuals. Am J Addict 1993;2(3):202–6.
40. Deykin EY, Buka SL, Zeena TH. Depressive illness among chemically dependent adolescents. Am J Psychiatry 1992;149:1341–7.
41. King C, Ghaziuddin N, McGovern L, et al. Predictors of comorbid alcohol and substance abuse in depressed adolescents. J Am Acad Child Adolesc Psychiatry 1996;35:743–51.
42. Schuckit MA. The clinical implications of primary diagnostic groups among alcoholics. Arch Gen Psychiatry 1985;1043–9.
43. Schuckit MA. Genetic and clinical implications of alcoholism and affective disorder. Am J Psychiatry 1986;143(2):140–7.
44. Schuckit MA. Alcohol and depression: a clinical perspective. Acta Psychiatr Scand 1994;377(Suppl):28–32.
45. Flory M. Psychiatric diagnosis in child and adolescent suicide. Arch Gen Psychiatry 1996;53(4):339–48.
46. Lewisohn PM, Hops H, Roberts RE, et al. Adolescent psychopathology I: prevalence and incidence of depression and other DSM-IIIR disorders in high school students. J Abnorm Psychol 1993;102:133–44.
47. Kandel DB, Raveis VH, Davies M. Suicidal ideation in adolescence: depression, substance use, and other risk factors. J Youth Adolesc 1991;20:289–309.

48. Rao U, Ryan ND, Dahl RE, et al. Factors associated with the development of substance use disorder in depressed adolescents. J Am Acad Child Adolesc Psychiatry 1999;38:1109–17.

49. Bukstein O, Kaminer T. The nosology of adolescent substance abuse. Am J Addict 1994;Winter:1–13.

50. Kaminer Y. Adolescent substance abuse: a comprehensive guide to theory and practice. New York: Plenum Medical Books; 1994.

51. Beck AT, Rush AJ, Shaw BF, et al. Cognitive therapy of depression. New York: Guilford Press; 1979.

52. Fishbein D, Novak SP, Krebs C, et al. The mediating effect of depressive symptoms on the relationship between traumatic childhood experiences and drug use initiation. Addict Behav 2011;36(5):527–31.

53. Riggs P, Levin F, Green AL, et al. Comorbid psychiatric and substance abuse disorders: recent treatment research. Subst Abus 2008;29(3):51–63. Review.

54. Riggs, PD, Lohman, M, Davies, R, et al. A randomized controlled trial of fluoxetine/placebo and CBT in depressed adolescents with substance use disorders. Abstract, Synposium presented at the 23rd Annual Meeting of the American Academy of Addiction Psychiatry. Scottsdale, Arizona, December 7–11, 2005.

55. Riggs PD, Mikulich-Gilbertson SK, Davies RD, et al. A randomized controlled trial of fluoxetine and cognitive behavioral therapy in adolescents with major depression, behavior problems, and substance use disorders. Arch Pediatr Adolesc Med 2007;161(11):1026–34.

56. Burke JD, Burke KC, Rae DS. Increased rates of drug abuse and dependence after onset of mood or anxiety disorders in adolescence. Hosp Community Psychiatry 1994;45(5):451–5.

57. Giaconia RM, Reinherz HZ, Silverman AB, et al. Ages of onset of psychiatric disorders in a community population of older adolescents. J Am Acad Child Adolesc Psychiatry 1994;33(5):706–17.

58. Riggs PD, Mikulich SC, Coffman L, et al. Fluoxetine in drug-dependent delinquents with major depression: an open trial. J Child Adolesc Psychopharmacol 1997;7:87–95.

59. Goldstein BI, Bukstein OG. Comorbid substance use disorders among youth with bipolar disorder: opportunities for early identification and prevention. J Clin Psychiatry 2010;71(3):348–58.

60. Wilens TE, Biederman J, Millstein RB, et al. Risk for substance use disorders in youths with child- and adolescent-onset bipolar disorder. J Am Acad Child Adolesc Psychiatry 1999;38:680–5.

61. Kaminer Y. Pharmacotherapy for adolescents with psychoactive substance use disorders. In: Rahdert E, Czechowicz D, editors. Adolescent substance abuse (NIDA research monograph 156). Rockville (MD): National Institute on Drug Abuse; 1995. p. 291–324.

62. Geller B, Cooper TB, Sun K, et al. Double-blind and placebo-controlled study of lithium for adolescent bipolar disorders with secondary substance dependency. J Am Acad Child Adolesc Psychiatry 1998;37:171–8.

63. Deykin EY, Buka SL. Prevalence and risk factors for posttraumatic stress disorder among chemically dependent adolescents. Am J Psychiatry 1997;154:752–7.

64. Kandel DB, Johnson JG, Bird HR, et al. Psychiatric comorbidity among adolescents with substance use disorders: findings from the MECA study. J Am Acad Child Adolesc Psychiatry 1999;38:693–9.

65. Clark DB, Bukstein O, Smith MG, et al. Identifying anxiety disorders in adolescents hospitalized for alcohol abuse and dependence. Psychiatr Serv 1995;46: 618–20.

66. Frojd S, Ranta K, Kaltiala-Heino R, et al. Associations of social phobia and general anxiety with alcohol and drug use in a community sample of adolescents. Alcohol Alcohol 2011;46(2):192–9.

67. Wilens T, Spencer T, Frazier J, et al. Psychopharmacology in children and adolescents. In: Ollendick T, Hersen M, editors. Handbook of child psychopathology. New York: Plenum Publishing; 1998. p. 603–36.

68. Wu P, Goodwin RD, Fuller C, et al. The relationship between anxiety disorders and substance use among adolescents in the community: specificity and gender differences. J Youth Adolesc 2010;39(2):177–88.

69. Clark DB, Lesnick L, Hegedus AM. Traumas and other adverse life events in adolescents with alcohol use and dependence. J Am Acad Child Adolesc Psychiatry 1997;36:1744–51.

70. Van Hasselt VB, Ammerman RT, Glancy LJ, et al. Maltreatment in psychiatrically hospitalized dually diagnosed adolescent substance abusers. J Am Acad Child Adolesc Psychiatry 1992;31(5):868–74.

71. Ford JD, Elhai JD, Connor DF, et al. Poly-victimization and risk of posttraumatic, depressive, and substance use disorders and involvement in delinquency in a national sample of adolescents. J Adolesc Health 2010;46(6):545–52.

72. Cohen JA, Mannarino AP, Zhitova AC, et al. Treating child abuse-related posttraumatic stress and comorbid substance abuse in adolescents. Child Abuse Negl 2003;27(12):1345–65.

73. Kelleher K, Chaffin M, Hollenberg J, et al. Alcohol and drug disorders among physically abusive and neglectful parents in a community-based sample. Am J Public Health 1994;84:1586–90.

74. Health and Human Services, Public Health Service, Substance Abuse and Mental Health Services Administration & Office of Applied Studies. National household survey on drug abuse: main findings, 1996. Rockville (MD): Substance Abuse and Mental Health Services Administration, Office of Applied Studies; 1998.

75. Murphy JM, Jellinew M, Quinn D, et al. Substance abuse and serious child maltreatment: prevalence, risk, and outcome in a court sample. Child Abuse Negl 1991;15:197–211.

76. Bays J. Substance abuse and child abuse—impact of addiction on the child. Pediatr Clin North Am 1990;37:881–904.

77. Bennett EM, Kemper KJ. Is abuse during childhood a risk factor for developing substance abuse problems as an adult? J Dev Behav Pediatr 1994;15:426–9.

78. Wells K. Substance abuse and child maltreatment. Pediatr Clin North Am 2009; 56(2):345–62.

79. Bateman DA, Heargarty MC. Passive freebase cocaine ("crack") inhalation in infants and toddlers. Am J Dis Child 1989;143:25–7.

80. Heidemann SM, Goetting MG. Passive inhalation of cocaine by infants. Henry Ford Hosp Med J 1990;38:252–4.

81. Mirchandani HG, Mirchandani IH, Hellman F, et al. Passive inhalation of freebase cocaine ("crack") smoke by infants. Arch Pathol Lab Med 1991;115:494–8.

82. Kintz P, Villain M, Dumestre-Toulet V, et al. Methadone as a chemical weapon— two fatal cases involving babies. Ther Drug Monit 2005;27(6):741–3.

83. Couper FJ, Chopra K, Pierre-Louis ML. Fatal methadone intoxication in an infant. Forensic Sci Int 2005;153:71–3.

84. Schwartz RH, Peary P, Mistretta D. Intoxication of young children with marijuana: a form of amusement for pot-smoking teenage girls. Am J Dis Child 1986; 140:326.

85. Wilens TE, Biederman J, Spencer TJ. Case study: adverse effects of smoking marijuana while receiving tricyclic antidepressants. J Am Acad Child Adolesc Psychiatry 1997;36:45–8.

86. Brown SA. Recovery patterns in adolescent substance abuse. In: Bae JS, Marlatt GA, McMahon RJ, editors. Addictive behaviors across the life span: prevention, treatment, and policy issues. Newbury Park (CA): Sage Publications; 1993. p. 161–83.

87. Hohman M, LeCroy CW. Predictors of adolescent AA affiliation. Adolescence 1996;31:339–52.

88. Simkin DR. Twelve-step treatment from a developmental perspective. Child Adolesc Psychiatr Clin N Am 1996;5:165–75.

The Impact of Food Insecurity on Child Health

Shilpa Pai, MD[a],*, Kandy Bahadur, MD[b]

KEYWORDS

- Food insecurity • Poverty • Child health

KEY POINTS

- Food insecurity is determined by multiple levels of diet impacts from the micro to the macro level.
- Because access to healthful and nutritious is one of the most fundamental needs of a child, lack thereof will lead to negative impacts on a child's health.
- By learning how to identify food insecurity, pediatricians can better address the overall well-being of a child.

INTRODUCTION

Food and satisfying hunger are at the base of Maslow's Hierarchy of Needs. Until food and hunger needs are met, humans cannot fulfill other higher-order needs. A food-insecure household is one in which "access to adequate food is limited by constrained resources."[1] Food insecurity is recognized as a public challenge both nationally and abroad. In 2017, 11.8% of United States households and 15.7% of households with children were food insecure at some point during the year.[1] Food-insecure children can manifest with many different ailments including hyperactivity, aggression, anxiety, depression, learning disabilities, and even frequent hospitalizations.[2–4] In addition, several studies noted that those children with food insecurity also had an increased prevalence of anemia,[5,6] hypercholesterolemia,[7] asthma,[8] hospitalization with diabetes,[9] physical inactivity[10] and overuse of medications.[9] For this reason, it is vital that pediatricians be aware of and screen for food insecurity in all patients.

BACKGROUND AND HISTORY

Although the concept of hunger was studied for some time, it was not until 1990 when a formal definition of food insecurity was decided on by a working group

[a] Department of Pediatrics, Rutgers-Robert Wood Johnson Medical School, 277 George Street, New Brunswick, NJ 08901, USA; [b] 720 US Route 202-206 North, Bridgewater, NJ 08807, USA
* Corresponding author.
E-mail address: paiss@rwjms.rutgers.edu
Twitter: @drshilpapai (S.P.)

Pediatr Clin N Am 67 (2020) 387–396
https://doi.org/10.1016/j.pcl.2019.12.004
pediatric.theclinics.com
0031-3955/20/© 2019 Elsevier Inc. All rights reserved.

for the American Institute of Nutrition in response to the National Nutrition Monitoring and Related Research Act.[11] The ability to measure and track food insecurity statistics allowed the United States Department of Health and Human Services to more accurately estimate and investigate the problems of hunger and malnutrition, which in turn allowed the development of key nutritional programs to combat food insecurity. Beginning in 1995, the Food Security Supplement, which includes the Household Food Security Survey Module (HFSSM), was added to the Current Population Survey sent to 60,000 households monthly to gain representative information on labor force characteristics. The HFSSM is a subset of 10 to 18 questions (depending on whether children are present in the household), in which the responses are used to calculate the food security scale and subsequent prevalence of food security.[12] Over time, the HFSSM has been analyzed and shortened to an even smaller subset of questions for various other research purposes while still keeping its sensitivity and validity.

EPIDEMIOLOGY

In the United States, rates of food insecurity increased significantly during the recession of 2007 to 2009. In 2007%, 11% of United States households were found to be food insecure. These rates peaked in 2011 at 14.9%. Since then, there has been a decline in the rates. However, food insecurity still exists across a wide distribution of United States households.

In 2018, the United States Department of Agriculture (USDA) reported that 13.9% of United States households with children younger than 18 years were found to be food insecure. Children are usually protected from decreases in a household's food intake—for example, caregivers may forgo their meals to ensure that their children have enough food to eat. Nonetheless, 0.6% of these households still had children who also experienced reduced food intake (**Fig. 1**).[1]

Of the households living with food insecurity, 13.9% included children, which is substantially higher than those food-insecure households without children (10%). In addition, married-couple families had the lowest rates of food insecurity (8.3%), whereas households headed by a single woman had the highest rates (29%). Regarding

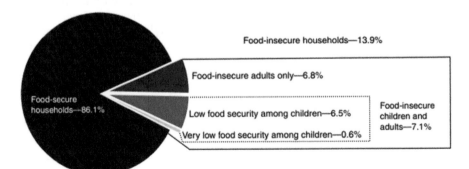

Fig. 1. United States households with children by food security status of adults and children, 2018. (*From* Coleman-Jensen A, Rabbitt MP, Gregory CA., et al. 2019. Household Food Security in the United States in 2018, ERR-270, U.S. Department of Agriculture, Economic Research Service Available at: https://www.ers.usda.gov/webdocs/publications/94849/err-270.pdf?v=963.1; and *Data from* U.S. Department of Commerce, U.S. Census Bureau, 2018 Current Population Survey Food Security Supplement. Available at: https://data.census.gov/mdat/.)

ethnicity, 21% of affected households were black and 16% Hispanic. Geographically, the highest rates of food insecurity were found in the southeastern United States, as well as those living in metropolitan areas.

Fig. 2, from the USDA, further delineates the prevalence of food insecurity among the various types of United States households in 2017 and 2018.

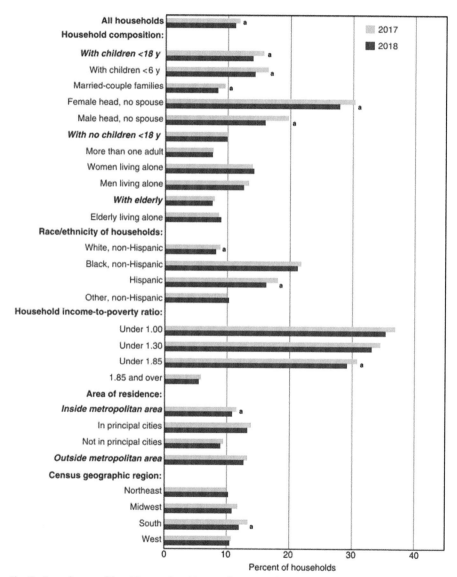

Fig. 2. Prevalence of food insecurity, 2017 and 2018. [a] Change from 2017 to 2018 was statistically significant with 90% confidence (t >1.645). (*From* Coleman-Jensen A, Rabbitt MP, Gregory CA., et al. 2019. Household Food Security in the United States in 2018, ERR-270, U.S. Department of Agriculture, Economic Research Service Available at: https://www.ers. usda.gov/webdocs/publications/94849/err-270.pdf?v=963.1; and *Data from* U.S. Department of Commerce, U.S. Census Bureau, 2018 Current Population Survey Food Security Supplement. Available at: https://data.census.gov/mdat/.)

The 2014 *Future of Children* research report, "Childhood food insecurity in the United States: trends, causes, and policy options," reported some other factors that predict children's food insecurity including mother's health, mother's substance abuse, residential instability, living in a household with both parents present, inconsistent child support payments, summertime, and immigrant parents.

CONTRIBUTORS TO FOOD INSECURITY

There are multiple levels of consideration when delving into the causes of food insecurity—from the individual to the social environment to the local environment and macroenvironment. At the individual level, one's eating habits are influenced by personal motivations, self-efficacy, outcome expectations, and behavioral capability. In a household where money for food is limited, choices tend to be based on taste and satiety rather than nutrient content, whereas the social environment will further affect food choices through the surrounding norms and supports. Parents may buy foods that they know their child will eat as opposed to spending their limited budget on trying something new and healthier, which their child may not eat. The physical environment plays a significant role because it is the setting where people eat and get food. It determines which foods are available and can be the barrier or opportunity that hinders or facilitates healthy eating. In addition, neighborhood characteristics may affect household food supply. For instance, food deserts may make it difficult for families to physically access healthy foods. Smaller, convenience-type stores may be more accessible and tend to carry the less healthful alternatives such as fresh produce, lean meats, and whole grains. Finally, the macroenvironment plays a more indirect role but will still have a substantial and powerful effect on what people eat. Owing to the complex forces of food marketing, food production/distribution, agricultural policies, and economic price structures, costs of nutrient-dense versus energy-dense foods are affected. For instance, the cost of nutrient-dense foods such as fruits, vegetables, and whole grains has increased faster than the cost of energy-dense foods (eg, chips and cookies). Recognizing the individual and the social environment, physical environment, and macroenvironment must be acknowledged when exploring the factors that influence a household's eating behaviors.[13]

IMPACT OF FOOD INSECURITY ON HEALTH AND WELL-BEING

The adverse health impacts of food insecurity are broad ranging, affecting a child's nutritional, physical, mental, and cognitive well-being. Beginning in utero, nutritional inadequacy can have long-lasting effects on cognitive and brain development that is affected by nutritional pathways.[14] A pregnant woman with poor quality of diet, limited quantity of food, yet higher nutrient demands heightens her own and her growing infant's risk of inadequate caloric and micronutrient intake. Food-insecure toddlers have a 140% higher likelihood of iron-deficiency anemia, which leads to impairments in cognitive, mental, and psychomotor development.[6] Adolescents have been found to have deficiency in protein, vitamin A, and magnesium.[15]

In one study, Alaimo and colleagues[16] found that preschool children in food-insufficient households had increased odds ratios for upper respiratory infections (1.57), stomachaches (3.0), and headaches (2.48) compared with their food-secure counterparts. In a separate study, Cook and colleagues[17] found children in food-insecure households to be 30% more likely to be hospitalized at least once since birth and 90% more likely to be in fair to poor health as opposed to good or excellent health.

Mental health is also altered by food insecurity. To begin with, mothers with food insecurity have a higher risk for depression, which can negatively affect the mother-child dyad.[18] Many times, depression coexists with substance abuse and domestic violence.[19] The finding that maternal mental health affects household food security is bolstered further by evidence from Noonan and colleagues, who used data from the Early Childhood Longitudinal Study Birth Cohort (ECLS-B). In this study, parents and caregivers (including early childhood teachers) of 14,000 children born in 2001 were interviewed 4 times between birth and the start of kindergarten. The investigators found that when mothers are moderately to severely depressed, the risk of child and household food insecurity increases by 50% to 80%, depending on the measure of insecurity. In addition, these mothers may lack energy to provide care, developmental stimulation, and consistent routines.[20] Consequently, this negatively affects parent-child interactions and attachment formation and may influence the risk of overweight toddlers.[21]

Food-insecure children will themselves experience mental health issues. They are more likely to demonstrate frustration, worry, and sadness about the food supply. Three-year-old children were found to exhibit behavioral problems such as aggression, inattention, irritability, and hyperactivity as measured on the Child Behavior Checklist. Preschool and school-age children had increased internalizing problems—experiencing more headaches, irritability, aggressiveness, hyperactivity, and stomachaches—which may be coping strategies.[13,18,22–24] Meanwhile, teenagers with food insecurity are 4 times more likely to have dysthymia, 5 times more likely to have attempted suicide, more likely to be depressed, and more likely to use mental health services and special counseling.[25]

Food insecurity will also affect a child's school readiness and performance. Caregivers from food-insecure households were found to be 66% more likely to report children at risk in expressive and receptive language, fine and gross motor movements, behavior, social/emotional development, self-help, and school performance.[26] Whereas kindergartners had impaired academic performance in reading, math, and social skills, school-age children were more likely to have repeated a grade, with lower math scores and higher rates of absenteeism, tardiness, and school suspension.[16,27]

ROLE OF THE PEDIATRICIAN

In the first 5 years of life, nutrition plays an essential role in cognition and problem solving, and it is during this period when children are at particular risk for the consequences of food insecurity. During this critical time, pediatricians are given at least 12 different opportunities during the multitude of well-child visits to screen for and intervene for food insecurity at each of the scheduled well visits as recommended by the American Academy of Pediatrics (AAP). These opportunities place pediatricians at the forefront for not only mitigating the effects of food insecurity by intervening, but also for identifying food insecurity as a potential underlying cause of other important physical ailments. To do so, pediatricians must be aware of evidence-based food insecurity screening practices as well as resources available.[28] Pediatricians' awareness on this matter is important to not only instruct parents on eligible nutritional resources but, more importantly, to have continuous follow-up with parents given the cyclic nature of food insecurity. Although there is no consensus on how often the follow-up should be, it should be regular enough that families have the opportunity to use the resources to determine benefits while at the same time not overburdening the practitioners. One way to mitigate the stigma of families having to ask for assistance is to have food insecurity informational posters that list local and federal nutritional programs available with hours of operation and qualifications in all examination rooms. Pediatricians should also have knowledge of potential barriers that families may face in receiving benefits, such as lack of personal or public transportation, changes in employment that may alter federal nutrition benefits on a monthly basis, lack of child care, and lack of school meals when school is out for the summer. Determining whether these barriers exist at the beginning of the visit will allow for a more realistic plan of action.

PREVENTION AND MANAGEMENT

In December 2015 the AAP released a policy statement recommending that pediatricians engage in efforts to mitigate food insecurity, be aware of resources that can attenuate the effects of food insecurity, and know how to refer eligible families.[28] The recommendations suggested that screening be included as a standardized component of care during all well-child visits, owing to the cyclical nature of food insecurity. This uniformity ensures that the underlying causes of clinical presentations are addressed before prescribing treatment or medication regimens, which helps to treat and prevent illness, supports patients in chronic disease management, and promotes wellness. Addressing the issue directly is often the least expensive or invasive treatment of food insecurity and has the fewest side effects.

Indicators for hunger are often hidden. Persistent hunger can be subclinical throughout the life cycle and not readily identifiable by anthropometric or biochemical indices. Recognizing predictors of food insecurity can help health care providers identify problems that might affect a caregiver's ability to comply with clinical recommendations, such as having to make a choice between medication and food. In the absence of overt signs of hunger, the clinician must rely on initial impressions, past chart notes, and screening questions to help identify a household at risk for food insecurity.

Consequently, to identify young children and families who may need assistance, the AAP recommends screening using the validated, two-question Hunger Vital Sign, which identifies households as being at risk for food insecurity if either or both of the these statements is answered as "often true" or "sometimes true": (1) "Within the past 12 months we worried whether our food would run out before we got money to buy more"; or (2) "Within the past 12 months the food we bought just didn't last and we didn't have money to get more."[29]

These are a subset of questions from the HFSSM: Household Food Security Survey Module. The Hunger Vital Sign screening questions measure families' concerns about and access to food, in much the way health care providers check other key vital signs, such as pulse and blood pressure. In asking the question, there must be an established trust, which is critical around the issue of food insecurity and a family's ability to feed the children. Therefore, training those who will be asking the questions on the health consequences of food insecurity, childhood hunger, and the importance of screening is crucial to establishing a safe place to discuss the sensitive issues of food insecurity. Families need to know they will be treated with respect and dignity. Approaching the conversation with sensitivity can elicit more honest and accurate information regarding food status.

As with any screening tool, a provider must know what to do with a positive answer to the questions. In the instances where there is a positive answer to the Hunger Vital Signs questions, it is crucial that clinicians become familiar with both short-term and long-term resources. The short-term solutions are typically emergency food sites available in the community, such as food pantries and soup kitchens. In providing these resources, it is important to include hours of operation, food options, and any limits on the amount of food provided.

Long-term resources are available from numerous government-supported agencies. In 1963, President John F. Kennedy proposed expanding and making permanent a small pilot project called the Food Stamp Program (which was enshrined in law the following year). Fifty years later this program, now called the Supplemental Nutrition Assistance Program (SNAP), remains the leading component in the safety net against hunger, assisting 1 in 7 Americans at a cost of $80 billion per year. SNAP directly augments a household's resources available for purchasing food. Monthly benefits can be used at grocery stores, farmers' markets, and food retail outlets that accept SNAP. Prior research has suggested that SNAP leads to reductions in food insecurity.[30] The Children's Health Watch researchers assert that SNAP benefits can make a crucial difference in determining a child's health status and development. Moreover, a study by Perry and colleagues[31] in 2007 reported that young children who receive SNAP benefits are 26% less likely to be food insecure than eligible children not receiving SNAP benefits. SNAP benefits can also do more than simply provide food assistance. Qualifying households can also receive other important assistance that supports family economic stability. According to the Center on Budget and Policy Priorities report, economists consider SNAP one of the most effective forms of economic stimulus. Moody's Analytics estimates that in a weak economy, every dollar increase in SNAP benefits generates about $1.70 in economic activity.

Following the successful implementation of the Food Stamp Program, Congress passed the Child Nutrition Act of 1966, which expanded the National School Lunch Program (NSLP) and established both the School Breakfast Program (SBP) and Child and Adult Care Food Program. The Special Supplemental Nutrition Program for Women, Infants, and Children (WIC) was added permanently in 1975.[32]

The NSLP and the SBP offer free or reduced-price school meals in participating schools. The NSLP is a federal assistance program that operates in more than 100,000 public and nonprofit private schools across the United States. At participating schools, children from families with incomes at or below 130% of the poverty level are eligible for free meals. According to the USDA Food and Nutrition Service Childhood Nutrition Guidelines of 2019 to 2020, children with household incomes between 130% and 185% of the Federal Poverty Level are eligible for reduced-price meals, which cannot cost more than 40 cents. The Community Eligibility Option allows schools in high-poverty areas to provide free breakfasts and lunches to all students if the percentage of households in the community participating in SNAP is high enough. If schools participate in the NSLP, the lunches they serve must meet certain federal requirements. No more than 30% of a lunch's calories may come from fat, with less than 10% from saturated fat. Lunches must also include at least one-third of the recommended dietary allowances of protein, vitamin A, vitamin C, iron, calcium, and calories.[32]

The SBP operates similarly to the NSLP. However, whereas almost all schools in the United States serve lunch, only 75% serve breakfast. This translates into 89,000 public schools, nonprofit private schools, and public and nonprofit private residential child care institutions that participate in the SBP.

WIC is another public health nutrition program designed to reach families most in need of preventive health services. WIC is federally funded and supported by the USDA. Those eligible for WIC include pregnant women, postpartum women, breastfeeding women, and children from birth to 5 years old. WIC clients receive nutritionally tailored monthly food packages, which they can redeem in grocery stores that accept WIC. The agency also provides breastfeeding support, nutrition services, health screenings, and provider referrals. In comparison with SNAP benefits, WIC vouchers can be redeemed at fewer outlets and for a much more limited set of foods.

Despite some families receiving the aforementioned nutrition assistance, many households, despite being eligible, do not. According to Feeding America research, only 41% of the households served by the Feeding America network report receiving SNAP benefits, although more than 88% are estimated to be income eligible. This suggests that many of the families who visit food pantries and meal programs are likely eligible but, for a variety of reasons, are not participating in the program.

Alternatively, the assistance a household receives may simply not be enough as benefits dwindle toward the end of the month. For example, SNAP benefits are not intended to cover all food expenditures. In other words, households receiving SNAP may be expected to spend some of their own income on food. Food-insecure families use diverse strategies to maintain food sufficiency. The Feeding America: Hunger in America, 2014 report shows that a caregiver may protect children from the full effect of inadequate food supply by purchasing inexpensive/unhealthy food (79%), receiving food from friends or family (53%), watering down food or drinks (40%), selling personal property (35%), or growing foods in gardens (23%). For this reason, it is vital to have regular follow-up of families who screen positive for food insecurity and to continuously assess for barriers to using resources, as well as assessing for changes in families' ability to qualify for certain resources.

ROLE OF TECHNOLOGY

There are several food insecurity screening tools available, including the18-item US Household Food Security Scale, the 2-item Hunger Vital Signs, and many iterations in between.[29] For a time-constrained office visit, a well-validated and practical option is the Hunger Vital Signs, which is recommended by the AAP.[28] There are several options for screening, including (1) having the parent or guardian complete the questions via paper or electronic device such as an electronic tablet while in the waiting room or (2) having the questions asked verbally by either the medical assistant or the physician. The questions can easily be integrated into the office's electronic medical records (EMR) in a location where physicians are already discussing nutrition and other risk factors, so as to increase ease and compliance with screening. As discussed earlier, it is important to have a referral guide for those families who screen positive for food insecurity. Whether the referral is a handout listing local and federal food-assistance programs or a referral to a social worker or community health worker, it can also be easily incorporated into the EMR. Lastly, there is an ICD-10 diagnosis code for food insecurity whereby physicians can more readily track these patients over time to (1) determine utilization or barriers to the use of recommended nutritional programs and (2) determine what additional help may be needed.

SUMMARY

Food insecurity has severe implications on children's health and their future. Children who are food insecure have a narrow bandwidth of food options, have limited access to healthy foods, and demonstrate poorer eating behaviors. The consequence of these coping strategies leads to chronic absenteeism, school failure, and chronic disease. Those with chronic disease will not only tend to contribute to higher health care expenditures but are more likely to become less employable as adults and, ultimately, to have lower household incomes. Although research has implied that food insecurity is inversely related to income, it is not synonymous with poverty because there are a significant number of families with income levels above the federal poverty level who still identify as being food insecure.[33] Therefore, it is prudent for pediatricians to screen universally. In addition, pediatricians should also advocate for protecting vital nutritional programs that exist to mitigate food insecurity, such as SNAP and WIC, and also advocate for increasing accessibility of nutritious, healthy food options, especially in locations labeled as food deserts. Given the severe implications of food insecurity, the collaboration of multidisciplinary teams including physicians, nutritionists/dieticians, and community health workers is necessary to facilitate enhanced care of all patients, especially those with food insecurity and other social determinants of health.

DISCLOSURE

The authors have nothing to disclose.

REFERENCES

1. Coleman-Jensen A, Rabbitt MP, Gregory CA, et al. Household food security in the United States in 2018, ERR-270, U.S. Department of Agriculture, Economic Research Service 2019. Available at: https://www.ers.usda.gov/webdocs/publications/94849/err-270.pdf?v=963.1.
2. Alaimo K, Olson C, Frongillo E, et al. Food insufficiency, family income, and health in US preschool and school-aged children. Am J Public Health 2000;91(5):781–6.
3. Casey P, Szeto K, Robbins J, et al. Child health-related quality of life and household food security. Archive Pediatr Adolesc Med 2005;159:51–6.
4. Ma C, Gee L, Kushel MB. Associations between instability and food insecurity with health care access in low-income children. Acad Pediatr 2007;8(1):50–7.
5. Park K, Kersey M, Geppert J, et al. Household food insecurity is a risk factor for iron-deficiency anaemia in a multi-ethnic, low-income sample of infants and toddlers. Public Health Nutr 2009;12(11):2120–9.
6. Skalicky A, Meyers AF, Adams WG, et al. Child food insecurity and iron deficiency anemia in low-income infants and toddlers in the United States. Matern Child Health J 2006;10(2):177–85.
7. Bahadur K, Pai S, Thoby E, et al. Frequency of food insecurity and associated health outcomes in pediatric patients at a federally qualified health center. J Community Health 2018;43(11):896–900.
8. Gundersen C, Ziliak JP. Food insecurity and health outcomes. Health Aff 2015; 34(11):1830–9.
9. Marjerrison S, Cummings EA, Glanville NT, et al. Prevalence and associations of food insecurity in children with diabetes mellitus. J Pediatr 2011;158(4):607–11.
10. To Q, Frongillo E, Gallegos D, et al. Household food insecurity is associated with less physical activity among children and adults in the U.S. J Nutr 2014;144(11): 1797–802.
11. Anderson S. Core indicators of nutritional state for difficult-to-sample populations. J Nutr 1990;120(11):1159–600.
12. Wunderlich GS, Norwood JK. History of the development of food insecurity and hunger measures. In: Panel to Review the U.S. Department of Agriculture's Measurement of Food Insecurity and Hunger, editor. Food insecurity and hunger in the United States: an assessment of the measure. Washington, DC: National Academies Press; 2006. p. 23–40.
13. Adams E. Childhood food insecurity. In: Oregon State University Professional and Continuing Education. 2008. Available at: https://pace.oregonstate.edu/courses/childhood-food-insecurity/food-access-and-food-cost/. Accessed July 22, 2019.

14. Abu-Saad K, Fraser D. Maternal nutrition and birth outcomes. Epidemiol Rev 2010;32:5–25.
15. Kirkpatrick SI, Tarasuk V. Food insecurity is associated with nutrient inadequacies among Canadian adults and adolescents. J Nutr 2008;138:604–12.
16. Alaimo K, Olson CM, Frongillo EA. Food insufficiency and American school-aged children's cognitive, academic and psychosocial development. Pediatrics 2001; 108(1):44–53.
17. Cook JT, Frank DA, Berkowitz C, et al. Food insecurity is associated with adverse health outcomes among human infants and toddlers. J Nutr 2004;134:1432–8.
18. Whitaker RC, Phillips SM, Orzol SM. Food insecurity and the risks of depression and anxiety in mothers and behavioral problems of their preschool-aged children. Pediatrics 2006;118(3):859–68.
19. Lawrence S, Chau M, Lennon MC. Depression, substance abuse, and domestic violence. New York, NY: National Center for Children and Poverty, Columbia University; 2004.
20. Huang L, Freed R. The spiraling effects of maternal depression on mothers, children, families and communities. Issue Brief #2. Baltimore, MD: Annie E. Casey Foundation; 2006.
21. Zaslow M, Bronte-Tinkew J, Capps R, et al. Food insecurity during infancy: implications for attachment and mental proficiency in toddlerhood. Matern Child Health J 2008;13:66–80.
22. Connell CL, Lofton KL, Yadrick K, et al. Children's experiences of food insecurity can assist in understanding its effect on their well-being. J Nutr 2005;135: 1683–90.
23. Kleinman RE, Murphy JM, Little M, et al. Hunger in children in the United States. Pediatrics 1998;101(1):e3.
24. Weinreb LC, Wehler J, Perloff J. Hunger: its impact on children's health and mental health. Pediatrics 2002;110:e41.
25. Alaimo K, Olson C, Frongillo E. Family food insufficiency, but not low family income, is positively associated with dysthymia and suicide symptoms in adolescents. J Nutr 2002;132(4):719–25.
26. Rose-Jacobs R, Black MM, Casey PH, et al. Household food insecurity: associations with at-risk infant and toddler development. Pediatrics 2008;121:65–72.
27. Jyoti DF, Frongillo EA, Jones SJ. Food insecurity affects school children's academic performance, weight gain, and social skills. J Nutr 2005;135:2831–9.
28. American Academy of Pediatrics Council on Community Pediatrics, Committee on Nutrition. Promoting food security for all children. Pediatrics 2015;136(5): e1431–8.
29. Hager E, Quigg A, Black M, et al. Development and validity of a 2-item screen to identify families at risk for food insecurity. Pediatrics 2010;126:E26–32.
30. Gundersen C, Oliveira V. The food stamp program and food insufficiency. Am J Agric Econ 2001;83(4):875–87.
31. Perry A, Ettinger de Cuba S, Cook J, et al. Food stamps as medicine: a new perspective on children's health. Children's Sentinel Nutrition Assessment Program; 2007.
32. Gundersen C, Ziliak J. Childhood food insecurity in the U.S.: trends, causes, and policy options. In: McLanahan S, editor. The future of children research report. Princeton-Brookings, Fall; 2014.
33. Gundersen C. Food insecurity is an ongoing national concern. Adv Nutr 2013; 4(1):36–41.

Supporting Children After School Shootings

David J. Schonfeld, MD[a,b,]*, Thomas Demaria, PhD[c]

KEYWORDS

• School • Shooting • Crisis • Bereavement • Adjustment • Coping

KEY POINTS

• There are a wide range of adjustment reactions that children may experience after a school shooting beyond trauma symptoms, even though many may not seem to be obvious to observers.
• Children (and adults) often feel guilt or shame associated with a school shooting, even when they have no objective reason to feel responsible.
• Pediatricians can play a critical role in helping children and their families cope after a school shooting.
• Pediatricians can advise schools on appropriate preparedness and response efforts and should recommend against high-intensity active shooter drills and the use of deception in live exercises.

INCIDENCE OF SCHOOL SHOOTINGS

A 2018 report from the US Department of Education and the US Department of Justice found that, from 2000 to 2017, there were 37 active shooter incidents at elementary and secondary schools and 15 active shooter incidents at postsecondary institutions. These school shootings resulted in a total of 153 casualties (67 killed and 86 wounded) in elementary and secondary schools, and 143 casualties (70 killed and 73 wounded) in postsecondary institutions in the 17-year period (2000–2017) studied.[1] Although these incidents receive high levels of media attention, school shootings are rare occurrences.[2] Even indirect exposure to traumatic events such as school shootings, including through communications from traditional and social media outlets, can heighten feelings of fear, anxiety, and vulnerability in children,[3,4] even if they did not attend the school where the shooting occurred.[5]

[a] National Center for School Crisis and Bereavement, Children's Hospital Los Angeles, 4650 Sunset Boulevard, #53, Los Angeles, CA 90027, USA; [b] Keck School of Medicine of the University of Southern California, Los Angeles, CA, USA; [c] National Center for School Crisis and Bereavement, Los Angeles, CA, USA
* Corresponding author. National Center for School Crisis and Bereavement, Children's Hospital Los Angeles, 4650 Sunset Boulevard, #53, Los Angeles, CA 90027.
E-mail address: schonfel@usc.edu

Pediatr Clin N Am 67 (2020) 397–411
https://doi.org/10.1016/j.pcl.2019.12.006
0031-3955/20/© 2019 Elsevier Inc. All rights reserved.

pediatric.theclinics.com

The National Institute of Justice[6] concluded that although violent crime at elementary, middle, and high schools in the United States actually decreased in recent years, the recent high-profile shootings at schools have led to the current perceptions about school safety and decisions to increase school security precautions, including increased use of armed security guards and police on school campuses, extensive use of security cameras, and high-intensity lockdown drills. These actions have been initiated despite limited evidence that these measures increase school safety, the substantial costs involved, and the possibility of causing emotional distress or discomfort in students and staff.

COMMON ADJUSTMENT REACTIONS SEEN IN CHILDREN

Most children who are experiencing adjustment difficulties after experiencing a school shooting may demonstrate no observable symptoms. This situation may mislead caregivers into believing that children were not affected by the event. Disruptive behavior patterns in children may even decrease in frequency following a school shooting owing to a large outpouring of social support and attention children receive.[7] Even children suffering from post-traumatic stress disorder (PTSD) may go undetected unless pediatricians and other pediatric health care providers (in this article, *pediatricians* will be used to signify pediatricians and other pediatric health care providers henceforth) screen or directly inquire about symptoms and adjustment. One of the core criteria of PTSD is an active avoidance of thinking about or talking about the triggering event and one's associated reactions to that event. Making the diagnostic process even more difficult, most of the symptoms of an acute stress disorder or PTSD may not be witnessed externally and not communicated by children to others (eg, intrusive thoughts, nightmares). As a result, parents, teachers, and other caregivers tend to underestimate the level of children's distress after a school shooting and overestimate their resilience, especially if relying on the observation of overt behaviors rather than inquiring specifically about feelings and reactions. The adults' own emotional reactions to the event also may diminish their ability to identify their children's needs if the parents' own emotional processing of the shooting takes precedence. For example, parents who are fixated on their own anger at who they believe to be responsible for the tragedy or parents who experience excessive guilt at not having protected their child may not be able to shift their personal focus from their own strong emotions to notice the subtlety of their child's emotional expressions. In addition, the parents' own difficulty adjusting to the school shooting may threaten children's sense of safety and security because children may believe their parents cannot protect them. Such parents also may serve as a negative model of emotional regulation.

Complicating the identification of adjustment problem is the tendency for children to use avoidance during difficult times. Children may want to spend even more time with their peers rather than parents and other adults and may therefore have less opportunity to express their feelings to adults. Children may also act immaturely at times of stress and become greatly concerned about themselves and disregard the feelings of others. Adults who do not understand this may see this as being selfish or uncaring and misinterpret this behavior as evidence that children are not impacted. It is important to make sure children feel comfortable in asking questions and expressing their feelings. Pediatricians can educate parents that they can expect their children to think more about themselves for the time being or not want to talk about what is bothering them. Once they feel reassured that they are being listened to and their needs will be met, children are more likely to be able to start to think about the needs of others as well as begin to express their own feelings, worries, and reactions.

Anticipatory guidance and advice can be provided by pediatricians to families on how to identify and address the most common adjustment reactions that can be anticipated among children after a school shooting that are outlined in **Table 1**.

The diagnostic criteria for PTSD[9] specify that a child or a family member must be exposed to actual or threatened death, serious injury or sexual violence and show evidence of persistent reactions for a least 1 month, including:

- Intrusive and unwanted memories, dreams, feelings, and detached (dissociative) play activity associated with the traumatic event often activated when the child is reminded of the event
- Avoidance of memories, thoughts, feelings, and external reminders (people, places, conversations, activities, situations) associated with the traumatic event
- Negative thoughts and feelings after the traumatic event including loss of interest in pleasurable solitary or social activities and blaming of self and/or others
- Change in arousal and reactivity associated with the traumatic event resulting in sleep difficulties, irritability, concentration problems, and hypervigilance

Distress after a school shooting often creates an additional burden for children with a prior history of traumatic exposure or adjustment difficulties.[10] Psychological issues that children have attempted to suppress may resurface, even if these issues are not directly related to the school shooting. As a result, unrelated events and experiences may be the cause for what seem to be reactions to the school shooting. In addition, future events and references that remind children of the losses or disturbing images, sensations, and emotions associated with the school shooting may serve as later triggers of their grief or trauma symptoms. News reports of another episode of community violence and discussions about similar mass shooting events on social media or in classroom lessons are common examples. These reminders may result in an unanticipated, acute resurgence of some of the feelings associated with the loss or crisis and catch children off guard. Pediatricians can advise children and their parents that they should anticipate that such triggers may occur so children can be helped to develop skills to anticipate and minimize triggers, as well as plan for how to address the associated feelings.[11]

RISK FACTORS FOR ADJUSTMENT DIFFICULTIES

The most vulnerable individuals in a school shooting event often include the primary victims (eg, those injured or threatened) or witnesses. As such, they should be offered psychosocial interventions even in the absence of visible distress.[12] Perceived support by the students from family and friends, however, seems to significantly decrease the risk of emotional difficulties.[10,13] This highlights the importance of increasing the support of students in their medical home.

The adjustment reactions of each individual child will also vary depending on a number of other factors, including:

- Personal connections or identification by the children with the shooting
- The duration of time before the children's daily environment, and that of the overall school community, returns to a safe, predictable, and comfortable routine (this return to a comfortable routine does not mean a return back to the baseline routine without needed supports and accommodations)
- The level of coping ability of the children's caregivers
- The children's preexisting mental health, developmental level, and baseline resiliency and coping/emotional regulation skills
- The nature of the secondary stressors, changes (eg, radical changes in school safety procedures) and losses that follow the school shooting

Table 1
Common symptoms of adjustment reactions after a school shooting

Symptom	Description	Comments
Sleep problems	Difficulty falling or staying asleep Frequent night awakenings or difficulty awakening in the morning Nightmares Other sleep disruptions	New sleep associations to cope with stress (eg, sleeping in a parent's bedroom) may be difficult to later modify
Eating problems	Loss of appetite Increased eating	—
Sadness or depression	—	May result in a reluctance to engage in previously enjoyed activities or a withdrawal from peers and adults
Anxiety, worries, or fears	Concern about repetition of traumatic event Increase in seemingly unrelated fears (eg, fear of dark when shooting happened during daytime) Separation anxiety or school avoidance	Students should return as soon as practical to a school-like setting (even if not to the same classroom or school) with accommodations and supports. Instead of requesting home-based education for a student with school avoidance, pediatricians should partner with the school to facilitate a transition back to school.
Difficulties in concentration	Difficulty learning or retaining new information Other difficulties progressing academically	A recent study of post-shooting student performance[8] found that school shootings dramatically decreased math and English scores on standardized tests.
Substance abuse	New onset or exacerbation of alcohol, tobacco, or other substance use	—
Risk-taking behavior	Increased sexual behavior or other reactive risk-taking	Seen especially among older children and adolescents
Somatization	Pains, fatigue, or other physical symptoms suggesting a physical condition	—

Developmental or social regression	Clinginess in young children Impatience Intolerance of change Irritability Disruptive behavior	—
Posttraumatic stress reactions	—	Posttraumatic stress or Acute Stress reactions are frequently observed immediately after and for weeks following traumatic events

BEREAVEMENT, SECONDARY STRESSORS, AND OTHER IMPACTS BEYOND TRAUMA

Whereas the adjustment difficulties that children experience after a school shooting may be related to posttraumatic reactions, many will not be directly attributable to the school shooting itself. The threat to life caused by a school shooting may worsen preexisting problems, such as an adolescent's increasing anxiety about the future after graduation or a child's feelings of helplessness related to bullying at school. Pediatricians may observe secondary losses and new stressors that may become the primary concern for a particular child or family. For example, schools that have experienced a shooting may experience a drop in enrollment, which has a negative impact on the school's budget. If this were to result in the discontinuation of an afterschool program that provided critical support or a sense of belonging to a particular student, that student may be reacting to the loss of the program in addition to, or even beyond, the personal impact of the shooting itself.

The management of these concerns requires a different approach than trauma treatment; pediatricians need to adopt a more holistic approach to assessing adjustment and promoting coping and resiliency among children and families after a school shooting. Assessments need not only to explore how children are adjusting with the shooting itself, but also to seek information about their current life circumstances and how they are dealing with the challenges these new circumstances may pose. Given that children may withhold voicing their concerns in the presence of their parents or other family members so as not to further burden the adults who may be in distress themselves, it is important for the pediatrician to interview children alone with the parents' permission and the children's assent when trying to assess fully their level of coping. Given that these secondary losses and stressors may continue or further develop for even several years after a school shooting, children's adjustment difficulties may persist for a similarly extended time.

If children experience the death of school staff or friends as a result of the school shooting, bereavement may emerge as their predominant concern. Pediatricians can serve as a useful resource for children who have recently experienced the death of a close family member or friend by helping their caregivers to understand the importance of inviting and answering their questions, providing information to help guide them in understanding and adjusting to the loss, and helping them to identify strategies for coping with the associated distress. Timely information about how to involve children in the funeral or other memorialization activities, how to enlist the support of school personnel, and bereavement support services available within the community are helpful to provide, through in-person meetings, phone calls, or psychoeducational materials.[11]

APPROACHES FOR PROMOTING COPING STRATEGIES

Advocating specific coping strategies for children after a school shooting can be challenging because of the interaction among a number of factors, including a child's personal characteristics and preferences, preexisting functioning, and developmental level at the time of the traumatic exposure. Research on stress management[14] has demonstrated that actively facing a problem is associated with better outcomes, and avoiding the situation or only reacting emotionally can be more problematic, although outcomes may vary depending on the nature of the stressors. Active coping may be most beneficial when stressors can be controlled by the child. Passive coping might be more productive when stressors cannot be readily removed. There are developmental progressions in the types of coping styles children use. For example, starting at ages 9 to 11, children begin to prefer using more active coping strategies.[15] Pediatricians can share with children that there are a variety of ways they can cope with stress[16] and encourage them to expand the coping strategies they use, which can make them more able to manage the different stressors they face.

Safety in the school setting can never be fully guaranteed, despite whatever actions a school may take after a shooting. Concerns and reactions among children and adults may increase in response to a reminder of continuing vulnerability, such as after a school shooting is reported in the news or when a school lockdown occurs because of criminal activity near the school, or even when due to a planned drill. Pediatricians should encourage changes that provide students with both physical, as well as psychological perceptions of, increased safety but that avoid overly restrictive measures (eg, armed guards and metal detectors) that can undermine the learning environment. The goal is to combine reasonable physical security measures (eg, locked doors and monitored public spaces, or asking teachers to stand in class doorways as classes dismiss for the period) with efforts to enhance school climate, build trusting relationships, and encourage students and adults to report potential threats.[17] After a school shooting, there will be students, staff, and families that adamantly seek more restrictive measures at the same time that others report that such restrictive measures are unneeded and serve as unwanted reminders of the school shooting and only cause many to feel more in danger.

Pediatricians can advise parents that telling children not to be worried is usually ineffective and undermines the potential for children to own their feelings and learn strategies to deal with them. If parents can also communicate some of their own worries, with an emphasis on sharing personal strategies they have used to cope effectively with those concerns, they provide opportunities for children to learn coping strategies. Families can also provide examples of additional coping strategies and model emotional regulation and a positive perspective.

Children (and adults) often feel guilt or shame associated with the school shooting, even when they have no objective reason to feel responsible. For example, children may feel guilty about their behavior during the event and fail to take into account that they responded automatically during a time of great danger. Children may also feel guilt, or blame others, as a way to feel some control over future traumatic events. If there was something that they did or failed to do that was responsible for the event in their mind, then they can reassure themselves that if they ensure that they do not repeat this mistake, another tragedy should not occur.

Psychotropic medications should generally be avoided in the short-term management of children's distress after a school shooting. Children need to process their memories, develop an understanding of the event, and learn to express and cope with their emotional reactions. Medication should, therefore, not be used to suppress reactions such as crying or feelings such as sadness and should not be used to blunt children's awareness. Referral to or consultation with a child mental health professional with expertise in the management of childhood trauma and loss is recommended for primary care providers when considering the use of psychotropic medications for persistent or severe posttraumatic reactions including self-injurious or dissociative episodes.

POTENTIAL ROLES FOR PEDIATRICIANS
Supporting Children in the Practice Setting

Pediatricians not only have a good understanding of the impact of trauma and loss on children and an appreciation of child development, but may also be uniquely positioned to both identify and address the concerns of children after such events. After tragic events, parents and other caregivers often hide their own distress to protect their children or provide them false reassurance; they may intentionally or unintentionally imply that children should not be upset.[18] Children in turn withhold their concerns so as not to burden adults who are visibly upset. Teachers and other school staff are likely as impacted to at least the same degree as students by a school shooting and may be so overwhelmed themselves that they are unable to appreciate adjustment difficulties in their students.

After a school shooting, pediatricians should raise the topic with all children involved, no matter how young they are.[10] Even children who have no direct connections with victims or other members of the school community involved in the shooting may nonetheless feel a sense of vulnerability when hearing about the shooting. Understanding more about a school shooting and how to cope with associated worries and reactions can help them better adjust. The National Center for School Crisis and Bereavement (www.schoolcrisiscenter.org) offers a free guidance document about how to talk to children about school shootings and terrorist attacks in the news (https://www.schoolcrisiscenter.org/resources/talking-kids-about-tragedies/).

The goals of short-term interventions after a school shooting are to address immediate physical needs and to keep children safe and protected from additional harm; to help children understand and begin to accept the traumatic event; to identify, express, validate, and cope with their feelings and reactions; to reestablish a sense of safety through routines and family connections; to start to regain a sense of mastery and control over their life; and to return to school and other developmentally appropriate activities. Older children will want and will benefit from more details and to discuss the larger implications of the event. Adults should provide reassurance that our government, police, and schools are taking steps to protect students from something like this happening again and to keep children safe. It may be helpful to clarify the actual low risk of a school shooting, which will likely seem far greater in the aftermath of a recent shooting.

Children who were wounded during the shooting will be brought to local pediatricians for after-care of their physical wounds. Children and their parents should be explicitly told that their visits can also be a time to address emotional recovery. Children who are grieving the loss of a family member or friend may benefit from bereavement counseling or support. Those experiencing or at high risk of developing PTSD (eg, children who directly witnessed the event, were wounded, or experienced dissociation at the time of the event) should be offered referral to a mental health professional experienced in cognitive-behavioral therapy that addresses trauma. Children with multiple stressors and/or chronic and ongoing trauma and those with limited external supports within their family, school, and broader community are more likely to require counseling or other formal support.

Even when it is obvious that there is nothing children could have done to prevent or minimize the crisis, students in the school may still feel helpless and wish they could have changed what happened. Pediatricians can let children know that this is a common reaction; we all wish that there is something we could have done to prevent a tragedy. Instead, suggest that together you can concentrate on what can be done now to help those most directly affected and to promote safety, tolerance, and acceptance in our communities.

The pediatrician can also explain that blaming others (eg, police, school) for not preventing the school shooting may be an attempt to regain control of uncomfortable feelings and a sense of personal risk. Blaming, however, does not decrease immediate feelings of grief and fear, nor does it provide any solutions for the future. Children should be told that, although it is common to feel angry, those that commit violent acts do not represent a particular racial, ethnic, religious, or other group. Children who are part of the same racial, ethnic, religious, or other group as the perpetrators of the school shooting may in turn worry that they will be targeted by others because of this perceived association and benefit from support from their pediatrician to address and cope with these concerns.

Sharing Strategies with Caregivers to Provide Support

Parents can be reminded by the pediatrician about how their own emotional reactions to the school shooting will often influence how their children process this event. Parents whose children survived a life-threatening situation will often be coping with a variety of emotions, including anxiety, anger, and guilt themselves. Parental trust in others, including school leadership, community leadership, and law enforcement, is often shaken. Seeing their children upset because of a traumatic exposure may engender feelings of parental guilt for not having protected their children. Having their children return to school may therefore be quite a challenge for the parents themselves as they struggle with the knowledge that it is impossible for the school to be totally safe. Parents may thereby inadvertently promote school avoidance in their children.

After a school shooting, parents will be worried about the ongoing emotional adjustment of their children and will often ask about warning signs they should monitor. The pediatrician can assure parents that children may continue to be very upset for several weeks after the shooting, but that most of these reactions will gradually dissipate in several months. Parents can be directed to call their pediatrician if the child or adolescent:

- Is unable to stop thinking about the shooting
- Shares any thoughts or gestures about harming self or others
- Displays any signs of substance use
- Is having trouble functioning in school, at home, or with their friends
- Is worried about other distressing experiences that have been triggered by the shooting

Pediatricians can remind parents that they should not wait until they think their child is in crisis. Parents should take advantage of counseling and support whenever they see significant distress.

Management of Media Interest

Exposure to media coverage of a tragedy often will increase anxiety in children even if they were not directly exposed to a school shooting.[19] Pediatricians can suggest to parents that they limit the amount of media coverage in the immediate aftermath of a school shooting for children and all members of the family, including television, radio, Internet, and social media, and remember that children often overhear and pick up on media coverage being viewed by adults. If media coverage is going to be viewed by children, parents can be encouraged to record and view it first and/or watch along with children. In discussions, parents should be encouraged to avoid graphic details and excessive information that is not helpful to understand what has happened or learn what to do to keep safe or to cope. If no further understanding is resulting from continued viewing of coverage of the event, then it is best for both children and adults to discontinue such viewing. Parents can be reminded that turning off electronic devices that are being used for entertainment may provide valuable time for the family to be together and provide support to one another after a school shooting. Providing this sense of belonging and connectedness can provide children more assurance that they will not be alone during the recovery process.

Public interest and media attention after a school shooting can be overwhelming. There can be a potential positive role for victims of a school shooting by engaging in advocacy efforts involving the media, but there are also potential negative impacts including provocative negative comments (trolling) and even death threats directed at children. Pediatricians should advise parents that being approached by journalists and being interviewed by the media can have a significant negative effect on posttraumatic distress in traumatized adolescents.[20] The pediatrician can also warn parents that some members of the media may reach out to children directly through social media to request comments or interviews and may coerce them by implying that real friends would agree to speak on behalf of their friends who were victims. Children should be directed to speak to their parents or other trusted adults before responding to such requests.

Serving as a Consultant to the School System

There are a variety of important ways in which pediatricians can assist schools in recovery efforts after a school shooting.

a. Children are helped by returning to their routine, such as school, organized activities, and sports, as soon as practical after a school shooting, as long as the necessary support systems and accommodations (such as temporarily decreasing or providing more time for homework assignments or tests) are in place. Pediatricians can suggest to schools that expectations for children's classroom performance and behavior should be modified until their adjustment difficulties no longer interfere with their cognitive, emotional, and social functioning. Parents and educators may be falsely reassured, however, by a return to routine, misinterpreting that children are more resilient than they may actually be and are no longer in need of support or assistance once they have begun the process of recovery. Children often need ongoing support for months or longer after a major tragedy, and some will require more intensive interventions. If supports and assistance are withdrawn before full recovery has occurred, some children will fail to return to their baseline level of adjustment and coping and may show continued impairment for an extended period of time.

b. After a school shooting, schools are likely to see negative effects on learning among their students. Teachers may find it difficult to teach or manage their classes unless adequate supports are put in place immediately after the school shooting and maintained until recovery has been completed.

c. Pediatricians can suggest to schools that, in addition to mental health services, schools can also provide opportunities for students to help others as they and other nearby schools recover from the school shooting and its aftermath. Having the opportunity to help others often assists in the adjustment and coping of the students providing such assistance.

d. Pediatricians can help schools to identify appropriate mechanisms for memorialization and commemoration. These activities provide a means for expressing grief and loss in a shared fashion, thereby decreasing isolation and promoting cohesion. When deaths have occurred as a result of a school shooting, these means of remembrance can reaffirm the personal attachment to the individuals who died and reassure the bereaved that loved ones will be remembered. Pediatricians can advise schools that such activities should involve the active participation of children and adolescents both in the planning and implementation to ensure that they are developmentally appropriate and personally relevant for them.[11,18]

e. Especially at the time of the 1-year mark of the shooting, schools and pediatricians can help children in their practice to shift the focus from the day of the tragedy to memories about the students and staff who died. Pediatricians can ask students in their practice if they have any specific personal memories that they feel comfortable sharing about a person who died that day.

Pediatricians can assist schools through guidance about the:

- Development of a reasonable timeline for emotional recovery for students and staff
- Emotional, physical, and behavioral signs of traumatic stress
- Range of coping strategies that can be used to foster resiliency
- Support for students with special needs
- Community and parent education materials
- Identification of students most likely in need of additional support
- Identification of staff who are most likely impacted themselves and strategies for these staff to obtain appropriate support

Advising on Preparedness Efforts

Pediatricians can work with schools before a tragic event occurs in a number of ways, including:

a. The development of policies and procedures that create a school climate that not only addresses potential security threats, but also fosters an environment where the unique needs of all children can be supported. "A Framework for Safe and Successful Schools"[17] was developed by 6 leading educational organizations and provides examples of "school safety policies that will genuinely support the well-being and learning of students over the long term, rather than reactive strategies that may cause more harm than good."

b. Advising schools that adopting school shooting media portrayals for profiling of students in school policies and procedures can contribute to dehumanization and subsequent negative attitudes toward children with emotional and conduct problems.[21] For example, a depressed and isolated teenager who dresses in unusual clothing may become the target for bullying by peers and avoidance by teachers who fear the student has a proclivity for violence.

c. Advocating for policies related to drills and exercises that are appropriate. This measure will require the pediatrician to be familiar with what drills are required by the state as well as the local practices, especially related to active shooter and other armed assailant drills. Nearly all of today's schools engage in lockdown drills.[22]

Student learning is promoted by a predictable school day and by perceptions that the school is a safe place.[23] Schools remain among the safest environments for children and youth, and incidents of armed assailants in schools resulting in injury or death are still quite rare. Many recognize the value of preparedness and remain concerned about the increase in such incidents. This has even resulted in the use of active shooter drills where deception is involved, wherein the students and staff are not informed that the situation is a drill and instead led to believe that it is a real event. This approach is based on the belief that the element of surprise and fear best prepares students and staff members to take the most appropriate actions during a real attack.

Given the rarity of actual attacks in schools and the practical and ethical barriers to empirically evaluating whether deception and associated fear would mitigate any mortality or morbidity in a real event, the evidence to support this view is lacking. Even if there is no deception and notice is given of a drill, it is likely that high-intensity drills, such as simulations involving theatrical makeup to represent gunshot wounds, gunfire or the use of blanks, and predatory acting by the mock shooter, may still be highly traumatic for children, especially those exposed to prior violence.

Participation in live drills and mock funerals (wherein students role play the aftermath of imagined student deaths, which may be seen when schools are attempting to increase fears of drinking and driving), even when participants are fully informed, is likely to cause significant distress and psychological harm for some participants. Negative responses may become exacerbated among those with prior losses or trauma, anxiety or stress disorders, or other behavioral health problems.[24] There is no evidence that simulated exercises that are highly distressing, such as those involving deception, are superior to other forms of drills for which students and staff members are aware they are being trained.

With any drill, pediatricians can serve as a valuable resource for guidance about accommodations based on a variety of factors, which can influence children's experience including:

- Age and developmental levels
- Disabilities that might impede mobility and access to instructions
- Neurodevelopmental disabilities such as autism that might heighten a distress reaction and/or impede response to instruction
- Intellectual disabilities that might impede understanding a situation or instructions
- Trauma history of children that may make the experience more frightening[23]

Lockout drills are generally less disruptive and stressful than the full-scale lockdown. Lockdown drills implemented effectively have been found to increase knowledge and skills of how to respond appropriately without necessarily elevating anxiety or perceived safety risk,[25] but there is no empirical research at this time supporting school-based armed assailant drills.[26]

Pediatricians should partner with school mental health clinicians and school administrators to ensure that policies are created that explicitly prohibit using deception in live crisis drills and mock death notifications (wherein children are notified about the death of students who have not in fact died, such as due to driving while under the influence) in school settings. At the local level, pediatricians can request the current policies of the school districts in their communities and inquire about practices related to simulations and drills. At the state level, they can advocate that any legislation requiring school active shooter drills should follow best practice guidelines, such as those from the National Association of School Psychologists and the National Association of School Resource Officers.[26]

Unique Setting of Communities Characterized by Chronic Violence and Cumulative Loss

In neighborhoods characterized by chronic community violence, such as frequent gang violence, children often suffer from cumulative trauma and loss. Poverty, discrimination, and neighborhood disorganization may intensify their grief reactions and hamper their adjustment. Children may demonstrate personal resiliency in dealing with their exposure to traumatic events to some extent, but often lack sufficient external support to cope effectively with serious trauma or death. Children do not get used to the death of their peers or family members. With each subsequent death, children may instead become sensitized to future losses. Children in these communities may come to believe that adults are unable to protect them and establish a safe environment. Children may turn to peers for support and engage in a range of risky behaviors to challenge their fears about their own mortality. This disappointment in caregivers may generalize to all adults, resulting in children becoming skeptical about any support or guidance provided by their school, faith-based leaders, and/or pediatricians. In working with these children, pediatricians should first focus on building a trusting relationship. This goal can be accomplished by asking children how the pediatrician can assist them to feel less vulnerable and establish more safety in their life. Often times this may be challenging because the pediatrician will not be able to change the environment where these children live. The pediatrician, however, can promise children that they can always express their concerns in their medical home and offer linkages to reliable community support systems.

IMPORTANCE OF PROFESSIONAL SELF-CARE

Working with children after an unimaginable event like a school shooting can be quite distressing and lead to vicarious traumatization or compassion fatigue. Pediatricians may also have had a relationship with students and staff who died during the tragedy, resulting in the pediatrician experiencing their own grief. The importance of always practicing self-care strategies in clinical practice becomes even more critical after a school shooting because of the increased emotional and social burdens pediatricians may experience. Developing a comprehensive plan for self-care should include the provision of time for the development of a professional support system, expansion of professional knowledge, balancing of personal and professional needs, increased personal awareness and a daily inclusion of activities that provide rejuvenation and revitalization.[27]

Providing continuous support to patients, their families, and others in the community after a school shooting can at times feel overwhelming. Pediatricians should remind themselves of the critical importance of making a positive lasting impact by supporting the development of resiliency in children and families and the positive contributions of their efforts to provide support and assistance. Pediatricians should couple this with conscious efforts to increase their own personal self-care and reduce compassion fatigue so that they can empathically attend to the needs and feelings of their patients as well as their own.

ON-LINE RESOURCES

For more resources:

- Visit www.schoolcrisiscenter.org, the website of the *National Center for School Crisis and Bereavement* (NCSCB), or contact the center at 1-877-536-2722.
- Visit www.grievingstudents.org, the website of the *Coalition to Support Grieving Students*.
- Visit www.aap.org/en-us/advocacy-and-policy/aap-health-initiatives/Children-and-Disasters/Pages/Promoting-Adjustment-and-Helping-Children-Cope.aspx, the American Academy of Pediatrics' Promoting Adjustment and Helping Children Cope resource page.

DISCLOSURE

The authors have nothing to disclose.

REFERENCES

1. Musu L, Zhang A, Wang K, et al. Indicators of school crime and safety: 2018. Washington, DC: National Center for Education Statistics, U.S. Department of Education, and Bureau of Justice Statistics, Office of Justice Programs, U.S. Department of Justice; 2019 (NCES 2019-047/NCJ 252571).

2. Shultz JM, Cohen AM, Muschert GW, et al. Fatal school shootings and the epidemiological context of firearm mortality in the United States. Disaster Health 2013; 1(2):84–101.

3. Furr JM, Comer JS, Edmunds JM, et al. Disasters and youth: a meta-analytic examination of posttraumatic stress. J Consult Clin Psychol 2010;78:765–80.

4. Eisenberg N, Silver RC. Growing up in the shadow of terrorism: youth in America after 9/11. Am Psychol 2011;66(6):468–81.

5. Brener ND, Simon TR, Anderson M, et al. Effect of the incident at Columbine on students' violence- and suicide-related behaviors. Am J Prev Med 2002;22(3): 146–50.

6. Carlton MP. Summary of school safety statistics: national institute of justice report, 2017. Washington, DC: U.S. Department of Justice; 2017. Available at: https://www.ncjrs.gov/pdffiles1/nij/250610.pdf.

7. Liao Y, Shonkoff ET, Barnett E, et al. Brief report: examining children's disruptive behavior in the wake of trauma – a two-piece growth curve model before and after a school shooting. J Adolesc 2015;44:219–23.

8. Beland LP, Kim D. The effect of high school shootings on schools and student performance. Educ Eval Policy Anal 2016;38(1):113–26.

9. American Psychiatric Association. Diagnostic and statistical manual of mental disorders. 5th edition. Washington, DC: Author; 2013.

10. Lowe SR, Galea S. The mental health consequences of mass shootings. Trauma Violence Abuse 2017;18(1):62–82.

11. Schonfeld DJ, Demaria T, Committee on Psychosocial Aspects of Child and Family Health, Disaster Preparedness Advisory Council. Supporting the grieving child and family. Pediatrics 2016;138(3):e20162147.

12. Norris F. Impact of mass shootings on survivors, families and communities. The national center for posttraumatic stress disorder. PTSD Research Quarterly 2007;18(3):1–7.

13. Suomalainen L, Haravuori H, Berg N, et al. A controlled follow-up study of adolescents exposed to a school shooting – psychological consequences after four months. Eur Psychiatry 2011;26(8):490–7.

14. Lazarus RS, Folkman S. Stress, appraisal and coping. New York: Springer; 1984.

15. Eschenbeck H, Kohlmann CW, Lohaus A. Gender differences in coping strategies in children and adolescents. J Indiv Differ 2007;28(1):18–26.

16. Ayers TS, Sandler IN, Bernzweig JA, et al. Handbook for the content analysis of children's coping responses. Tempe (AZ): Program for Prevention Research, Arizona State University; 1989.

17. Cowan KC, Vaillancourt K, Rossen E, et al. A framework for safe and successful schools [brief]. Bethesda (MD): National Association of School Psychologists; 2013.

18. Schonfeld D, Quackenbush M. The grieving student: a teacher's guide. Baltimore (MD): Brookes Publishing; 2010.

19. Holman EA, Garfin DR, Silver RC. Media's role in broadcasting acute stress following the Boston Marathon bombings. Proc Natl Acad Sci U S A 2014; 111(1):93–8.

20. Haravuori H, Suomalainen L, Berg N, et al. Effects of media exposure on adolescents traumatized in a school shooting. J Trauma Stress 2011;24(1):70–7.

21. O'Toole M, Fondacaro M. When school-shooting media fuels a retributive public: an examination of psychological mediators. Youth Violence Juv Justice 2017; 15(2):154–71.

22. U.S. Government Accountability Office. Emergency management: improved federal coordination could better assist K-12 schools prepare for emergencies. Washington, DC: Author; 2016.
23. National Association of School Psychologists. Mitigating negative psychological effects of school lockdowns: brief guidance for schools. Bethesda (MD): Author; 2018.
24. Schonfeld DJ, Rossen E, Woodard D. Deception in schools—when crisis preparedness efforts go too far. JAMA Pediatr 2017;171(11):1033–4.
25. Zhe EJ, Nickerson AB. Effects of an intruder crisis drill on children's knowledge, anxiety, and perceptions of school safety. Sch Psychol Rev 2007;36(3):501–8.
26. National Association of School Psychologists, National Association of School Resource Officers. Best practice considerations for schools in active shooter and other armed assailant drills. Bethesda (MD): National Association of School Psychologists; 2014.
27. Dorociak K, Rupert P, Bryant F, et al. Development of a self-care assessment for psychologists. J Couns Psychol 2017;64(3):325–34.

The Intersection of Child Trafficking and Health Care
Our Unique Role as Pediatric Clinicians

Nicole M. Leopardi, MD[a], Aldina M. Hovde, MSW[b],*,
Lauren V. Kullmann, BS[c]

KEYWORDS

- Human trafficking • Child trafficking • Adverse childhood experiences (ACEs)
- Labor trafficking • Sex trafficking
- Commercial sexual exploitation of children (CSEC) • Trauma-informed care
- Screening

KEY POINTS

- It is important to recognize the breadth and scope of sex and labor trafficking of children and its impact in the United States.
- Common societal myths and misconceptions about trafficking inform healthcare clinician biases.
- Healthcare clinicians should be aware of the barriers of trafficking victims to seek healthcare and disclose their trafficked status, and should recognize the importance of implementing a trauma-informed care model in clinical settings.
- There are various trafficking surveys and screening tools currently available for clinical use, but there are limitations to the applicability and practical use of these tools.

INTRODUCTION

Human trafficking is a public health issue, a violation of human rights, and a crime in every state of the United States. Human trafficking is also a global issue, having an impact on every nation throughout the world. The International Labour Organization estimates that there are approximately 40.3 million victims of human trafficking worldwide, generating an estimated $150 billion annually. They also estimate that

[a] Pediatrics Clerkship, Medical Home for Trafficked Minors, Cooper University Healthcare, Children's Regional Center, CMSRU, 3 Cooper Plaza, Suite 200, Camden, NJ 08103, USA; [b] Safety and Trauma Informed Care Initiatives, New Jersey Chapter, American Academy of Pediatrics, 50 Millstone Road, Building 200, Suite 130, East Windsor, NJ 08520, USA; [c] Rowan University, School of Osteopathic Medicine, 1 Medical Center Drive, Stratford, NJ 08084, USA
* Corresponding author.
E-mail address: ahovde@njaap.org

Pediatr Clin N Am 67 (2020) 413–423
https://doi.org/10.1016/j.pcl.2019.12.005
0031-3955/20/© 2019 Elsevier Inc. All rights reserved.

approximately 81% of victims are trapped in forced labor, 75% are female, and 25% are children.[1]

Human trafficking is considered a form of modern-day slavery, involving the use of force, fraud, and/or coercion for the purpose of sexual exploitation or forced labor.[2] "The federal Victims of Trafficking and Violence Protection Act of 2000 and its subsequent reauthorizations define human trafficking as

1. Sex trafficking in which a commercial sex act is induced by force, fraud, or coercion or in which the person induced to perform such act has not attained 18 years of age; or
2. The recruitment, harboring, transportation, provision, or obtaining of a person for labor or services, through the use of force, fraud, or coercion for the purpose of subjection to involuntary servitude, peonage, debt bondage, or slavery."[3]

The primary difference between labor and sex trafficking of children is that force, fraud, or coercion must be a component of child labor trafficking, whereas any child engaged in a commercial sex act with or without the use of force, fraud, or coercion is considered a sex trafficking victim.[4] Importantly, labor and sex trafficking of children may co-occur.[5]

While human trafficking has an impact on people of every background, race, ethnicity, and religion,[6] there are individual, societal, and environmental risk factors that make some individuals more vulnerable to trafficking than others. Specifically those individuals with adverse childhood experiences (ACEs) are much more vulnerable to becoming a victim of human trafficking.[7]

EPIDEMIOLOGY

Estimates regarding the rates of human trafficking, including the trafficking of children, vary widely[8] due to several factors, including the secretive nature of trafficking,[9] fear of violence or deportation,[10] varying definitions,[9,11] and lack of awareness and education about how to identify and respond to suspected cases of trafficking.[8,12] State laws also vary on reporting requirements and the type of abuse that is reportable.[13]

It thus remains a challenge to identify the true number of total victims of human trafficking in the United States; however, Polaris[1] estimates that the number of victims nationally likely reaches into the hundreds of thousands when both adults and minors as well as sex trafficking and labor trafficking are combined. According to the National Human Trafficking Hotline, in 2017 alone, more than 8700 cases of human trafficking were reported, of which 29% were minors and 82% were female.[14] Overall, slightly more human trafficking victims were US citizens/lawful permanent residents compared with foreign nationals. There currently are no reliable data about the average age of entry into trafficking; however, a common age of entry is thought to be around the start of puberty.[15] Most reported cases were identified as sex trafficking, with labor trafficking the second most common form reported. Child labor trafficking occurs in a variety of industries, including "agriculture, domestic work, health and beauty, restaurants/small businesses, gang-involved drug sales and gun carrying, traveling sales crews (eg, magazine sales), and peddling/begging rings."[16] Given the number of industries in which children can be labor trafficked, it often is difficult to identify them as victims, particularly if they do not appear to be under force, fraud, or coercion.

Although there is general agreement about the breadth of the problem, there remains a dearth of information, data, and research to fully illuminate the prevalence and trends both globally and locally. In 2016, the US Department of State released the "Trafficking in Persons Report,"[17] suggesting that through collaboration, public awareness, research, data collection, program evaluation, and policies and programs to reduce risk, commitments to the 3P paradigm—prosecution, protection, and prevention—can be achieved. Clinicians are in a unique position to have a meaningful impact on both the protection and prevention domains of the 3P paradigm, because it is likely that most health care clinicians unknowingly encounter trafficking victims in their practice and posses the resources to intervene.[18]

REPORTING CHALLENGES

Human trafficking is a multifaceted public health crisis and human rights violation that is both under-recognized and under-reported, enabling perpetrators to continue to exploit and manipulate children in a vicious cycle of abuse. The commercial sexual exploitation of children (CSEC), which includes sex trafficking, claims an estimated 200,000 pediatric victims per year in the Untied States.[16] Completely reliable statistics are lacking due to the absence of a unified reporting system as well as difficulties defining, responding to, and quantifying CSEC; thus, estimates likely only represent the tip of the iceberg.[19] State laws also vary on reporting requirements. Some states require the involvement of child protective services, whereas others require reports to law enforcement, or both.[15]

Additionally, there are many barriers to identifying these victims, including the tendency for trafficked children to inconsistently self-identify as victims. The formation of trauma-coerced attachments known as "trauma bonds" in the face of low self-esteem, homelessness, dysfunctional family life, and prior abuse, creates a false sense of autonomy for victims and leads to coerced dependence on their trafficker, or psychological entrapment. Trauma bonds create changes in a victim's worldview and contribute to poor insight into his or her status as a victim as well as increase risk for revictimization.[20,21]

OPPORTUNITIES FOR INTERVENTION

Trafficking victims seek medical care at a relatively high rate while being trafficked. It is therefore likely that most health care clinicians have unknowingly encountered trafficking victims during the course of their careers.[18] Trafficked youth interact with clinicians in mental health clinics, reproductive health offices, primary care offices, emergency departments, and substance abuse treatment centers while still under the control of their traffickers.[22] They often present with physical complaints, such as abdominal pain and back pain, body image concerns, reproductive and sexual health concerns, and mental health issues. Trafficking leads to these and variety of other health complaints, as noted by Greenbaum and colleagues, positing "healthcare providers in a unique position to help potential victims."[7]

Accordingly, health care clinicians benefit from comprehensive education that provides them with the tools to identify suspected victims. There are many red flags that indicate an individual is at a higher risk of victimization, as highlighted in **Table 1**.[7,14] Although the table is not exhaustive, it can serve as a starting point for clinicians.[14] For example, ACEs, including child abuse, neglect, and household dysfunction, are linked to an increased risk of becoming a victim of child trafficking. The effect of ACEs on a child's self-esteem and home life lead to increased susceptibility to coercion and manipulation and thus increased vulnerability to the recruitment and control tactics employed by traffickers. "Given the trauma they have endured, victims are vulnerable to recruiting techniques involving seduction, coercion, and promise of protection occurring at shopping malls, bus and train stations, and even schools."[23] In addition

Table 1
Potential red flags of all forms of human trafficking

History and Presentation	Behavior/Demeanor	Physical
• Delayed presentation	• Poor eye contact	• Branding or unusual tattoos, for example, names, initials, barcodes
• Presenting with a controlling adult, significant other, and/or "translator"	• Reluctant to speak	• Physical injuries, for example, bruises, fractures, bites, burns, ligature marks
• Inconsistent or "rehearsed" history	• Fearful, anxious, submissive, hypervigilant, or defensive demeanor	• Signs of deprivation, dehydration, and/or exhaustion
• History of abuse and/or neglect	• Overly modest	• Signs of malnourishment, stunted growth and/or development
• History of running away/homelessness	• Insecurities regarding body image	• Poor dentition and broken teeth
• Living in poverty	• Appearing older or younger than stated age	• Foreign material in the vaginal vault (ie cotton)
• Foster care status	• Expressing concerns regarding next meal or need for shelter	• Concern for sexually transmitted infections, especially recurrent sexually transmitted infections
• Involvement with juvenile justice	• Attachment to cell phone	
• Few personal possessions		
• Discordant, expensive accessories		
• Lack of identification and/or insurance		
• Frequent changes of address/moving		
• Unexplained school absences		
• History of suicide attempt(s)		
• History of substance abuse		
• Lack of interest in activities		
• High number of sexual partners (>5)		
• History of pregnancies and/or abortions		
• History of pelvic pain, urinary tract infections, sexually transmitted infections		

to ACEs, there are specific individual, societal, and environmental risk factors that increase vulnerability to trafficking, in particular homelessness and foster care placement. According to reports to the National Center for Missing and Exploited Children (NCMEC), in 2017 an estimated 1 out of 7 endangered runaways reported to NCMEC likely were child sex trafficking victims.[24] Of those, 88% were in the care of the child welfare system when they ran away.[24]

Youth with these risk factors could have possibly gone un-noticed by traffickers in the past but now are much more readily accessible due to the widespread use of different technologies, including social media, interactive video games, cell phone applications, and other online platforms. According to Polaris, "case data from January 2015 through December 2017 records 845 potential victims recruited on internet platforms. This includes: 250 potential victims recruited on Facebook, 120 recruited on a dating site, 78 recruited on Instagram, 489 recruited on another type of Internet platform such as Craigslist, chat rooms, or a website that could not be identified during the hotline call."[25]

RECOGNIZING SOCIETAL AND CLINICAL BIAS

Although understanding the red flags and potential indicators of child trafficking is crucial, it also is important to recognize that individual patients may present as healthy, thriving children. The following case scenarios describe several seemingly thriving adolescents presenting with evidence of the long-term physical, mental, and reproductive concerns that affect children who have been trafficked.

One patient, a 16-year-old girl, with a sweet disposition and a quiet voice, presents for her well visit. Her hair is dyed with streaks of bright color and she is concerned about chronic abdominal pain and intermittently depressed mood. At first glance she appears to be like many other teenagers in a typical pediatric practice, but she, like countless others, is a victim of human trafficking.

Another patient, a 14-year-old boy, presents for his well visit. He is talkative, outgoing, and friendly. He has moved a lot over the past few years, living in various states with various family members and he enjoys speaking about his travels. He, too, is a victim of human trafficking, one of the many male victims who may be underestimated in the available data.

The last patient is a 17-year-old girl who is bubbly and engaged. She describes a longstanding history of back pain and scoliosis that has not been fully addressed by doctors in the past. She also is worried about the appearance of her toenails and is interested in starting some form of birth control. Like the other patients, she has survived human trafficking.

These brief cases attempt to illustrate the theme that, although there are many red flags and risk factors, when assessing a child 1-on-1 in the office or clinic, clinicians must acknowledge their biases and consider the possibility of trafficking in all youth, or it will continue to be missed.

In further consideration of potential biases present in health care clinicians, it is first necessary to address the widespread societal attitudes and misconceptions about human trafficking. Although strides have been made and efforts to improve education are ongoing, there remains a distinct lack of awareness among those on the front lines as well as a lack of empathy toward the victims once identified. A tendency to judge and to stigmatize persists; for example, labeling sex trafficking victims as "prostitutes" rather than appropriately approaching them as traumatized victims. Researchers in Wisconsin surveyed a group of 168 health care clinicians to determine how they would classify the victims in various cases of sex trafficking; 10% of clinicians in the study labeled the child victim a prostitute rather than a sex trafficking victim. The investigators postulated that clinician responses likely reflect the societal belief that children involved in the sex trade are responsible for their victimization.[26] The findings in this study also reinforce the need for human trafficking education to help clinicians acknowledge these biases and arm themselves with the tools necessary to recognize and intervene in potential human trafficking cases.

Misconceptions and myths about trafficking likewise cloud clinical judgment and lead to missed opportunities. Victimized children are not exclusively found in other countries and are not all immigrants into the United States.[27] In fact, the United States is one of the largest markets for trafficking in the world and many victims are US citizens or lawful permanent residents.[28] Likewise, "within the United States, [...] victims come from all backgrounds, sexes, nations, and economic levels."[6] Children are vulnerable by definition, but child victims of human trafficking often have increased levels of vulnerability and thus increased risk due to a history of abuse, homeless and/or throwaway status, personal or parental history of substance abuse, and/or involvement with the foster care or juvenile justice systems.[23] Special consideration also should be given to children who identify as lesbian, gay, bisexual, transgender, and/or questioning as well as those with mental illness or cognitive impairment, because these factors also increase vulnerability to traffickers.[23]

Awareness of the risk factors and red flags of trafficking as well as implementation of a trauma-informed care approach in the clinical setting all have the potential to greatly improve the care of this population of patients. Dignity Health has developed the PEARR Tool in partnership with HEAL Trafficking and with the Pacific Survivor Center to aid health care clinicians in providing a trauma-informed approach for patients at high-risk of abuse, neglect, or violence.[29] The tool provides a brief overview of the risk factors, potential indicators, and resources related to child abuse and neglect, abuse and neglect of vulnerable adults, domestic violence, sexual violence, and human trafficking.[29]

In a study conducted by Barnert and colleagues,[22] unique factors that influence a victim of trafficking to engage with clinicians were explored. Study subjects consisted of 21 adult women who were trafficked as children. Through survey and semistructured 1-on-1 interviews, various themes emerged: (1) barriers to obtaining and engaging with health care include a victim's disconnect and distrust of providers and institutions, a significant fear of confidentiality breaches, a fear of being judged, and, in some circumstances, the challenges of seeing male clinicians; (2) conversely, clinician respect, flexibility, and a pattern of shared decision making, or choice, emerged as facilitators of seeking health care. Overall, this study demonstrated what the authors labeled a model of fierce autonomy, in which victims share an amplified will toward self-determination and firm commitment to ownership over decision making with the underlying theme of the importance of feeling safe in order to effectively communicate with clinicians.[22] Although this model easily could be applied to adolescent patients, other techniques may be needed when working with younger children. Beyond clinician characteristics, it also is important to recognize the many barriers that victims must overcome when considering disclosure; see **Table 2**[7,30] for a more comprehensive list of potential barriers.

The patient voice is especially relevant when delivering trauma-informed care to human trafficking victims. Corbett explored survivors' recommendations regarding factors that assisted with their successful exit from CSEC.[6] Health care clinicians who engaged in active listening and who displayed encouragement and empathy (including showing love, support, and hope) as well as a nonjudgmental approach successfully facilitated rather than hindered their exit. Survivors voiced the theme, "Don't leave when we push you away."[6] Shared decision making when delivering trauma-informed care confers agency and builds meaningful relationships between victims

Table 2
Barriers to disclosure

- Fear of being released back to the trafficker
- Fear of harm to themselves, coworkers, friends, or family members
- Fear of being sent back to a prior abusive environment
- Prior unsuccessful attempts to leave or escape
- Feeling overwhelmed or frightened
- Young age
- Stigma and shame
- Uncertainty regarding geographic location
- Language barriers combined with lack of availability of a trusted professional interpreter
- Physical or mental illness or disability
- Cultural or religious prohibitions against speaking up

- Sexual orientation or lifestyle
- Inability to speak privately with the health care clinician
- Unfamiliarity with the health care system
- Distrust of authority figures, including those in health care
- Prior negative experiences (self or peers) following attempts at disclosure or help-seeking
- Lack of money to pay for medical care
- Lack of safe options post-disclosure
- Fear of deportation
- Prior criminal record

and clinicians while simultaneously respecting patient preferences, providing patients with autonomy and basic human dignity.[7]

SCREENING AND DIAGNOSIS

When committing to a trauma-informed approach in the pediatric clinic, screening for trauma is always a component of the model. "Victims may be reluctant to disclose their victimization due to shame, fear of their trafficker, or fear that they will be arrested and prosecuted for prostitution."[26] In other cases, they may not even recognize that they are being trafficked. "Victims seldom self-identify and clinically validated screening tools for the healthcare setting are lacking."[7] Implementing universal screening for ACEs in general and/or for human trafficking in specific are both viable options. Although various survey tools are emerging and being researched, there currently are no universal screening tools for all forms of human trafficking that are

Box 1
Survey for sex trafficking

1. Has anyone ever asked you to have sex in exchange for something you wanted or needed (money/food/shelter/other items)?

2. Has anyone ever asked you to have sex with another person?

3. Has anyone ever taken sexual pictures of you or posted such pictures on the Internet?

Data from Greenbaum, J, Crawford-Jakubiak J and Committee on Child Abuse and Neglect. Child sex and commercial sexual exploitation: Healthcare needs of victims. *Pediatrics.* 2015; Vol 135 (3): 566574; with permission.

Box 2
Child sex trafficking screening tool

1. Have you ever broken any bones, had any cuts that required stitches, or been knocked unconscious?

2. Some kids have a hard time living at home and feel that they need to run away. Have you ever run away from home?

3. Kids often use drugs or drink alcohol, and different kids use different drugs. Have you used drugs or alcohol in the past 12 months?

4. Sometimes kids have been involved with the police. Maybe for running away, for breaking curfew, for shoplifting. There can be lots of different reasons. Have you ever had any problems with the police?

5. If you have had sex before, how many sexual partners have you had (0, 1–5, 6–10, <10)?

6. Have you ever had a sexually transmitted disease, like herpes or gonorrhea or chlamydia or trichomonas?

Scoring the questionnaire.

Positive answers to 2 or more questions is considered a positive screen (eg, high risk). However, further information will be needed to determine whether or not a child is actually being trafficked.

Question 5 is considered positive if child reports greater than 5 sexual partners.

Data from Greenbaum VJ, Livings MS, Lai BS, et al. Evaluation of a tool to identify child sex trafficking victims in multiple healthcare settings. J Adolesc Health. 2018 Dec;63(6):745-752. https://doi.org/10.1016/j.jadohealth.2018.06.032. Epub 2018 Oct 4.

---

clinically validated for use in the pediatric clinic setting. See **Box 1**[7] for a 3-question tool developed by Greenbaum and colleagues when surveying for sex trafficking. See **Box 2**[31] for a more recently developed 6-question screen tool published by Greenbaum and colleagues that may be useful in various pediatric settings to screen for risk of child sex trafficking. The National Institute of Justice has also developed a comprehensive Trafficking Victim Identification Tool, available in full and abbreviated versions, that screens for both sex trafficking and labor trafficking. Even the abbreviated version, however, is quite extensive and may only be a reasonable option for certain clinical settings.[32] Research to further identify validated universal human trafficking screening tools in pediatrics is ongoing; however, even in the absence of a universal screen, health care clinicians can still make a significant impact in their clinics and in the lives of victims through education and commitment to a trauma-informed care approach.

SUMMARY

Human trafficking is a public health crisis and human rights violation. Victims of trafficking are seen in every clinical setting and in every state. They will continue to represent missed opportunities until health care clinicians fully recognize their distinct role in actively identifying and intervening for these patients. Understanding the risk factors for victimization as well as the red flags seen in victims is the first step, but it is not enough. Each case of trafficking is unique and many patients present as otherwise healthy children. There may be only slight nuances in the history or physical that enable a clinician to consider and accurately diagnose a human trafficking victim.

The use of existing resources and the further development of validated universal screening tools in pediatrics are necessary given the many barriers to disclosure for these patients. Health care staff who have direct clinical contact with patients should be educated to recognize the signs of child trafficking as part of a trauma-informed care model. It is important that health care clinicians create a safe environment, build trust, and ask the right questions to facilitate a patient's ability to disclose a history of trafficking.

There are many next steps in this process, including the standard use of trauma-informed care models in health care settings, implementation of mandatory trafficking education for health care clinicians, creation of additional screening tools and validation for use in pediatric clinics, and finally the development of a unified pathway for reporting and quantifying cases with appropriate intervention resources in place for each state. By reducing vulnerabilities present in children and families through early identification of ACEs and other risk factors, health care clinicians can work to prevent all forms of trafficking and exploitation of children, ultimately decreasing both the risk of being trafficked as well as the risks that lead to becoming a perpetrator of violent crimes.

DISCLOSURE

The authors have nothing to disclose.

REFERENCES

1. Polaris. The facts. 2019. Available at: https://polarisproject.org/human-trafficking/facts. Accessed July 26, 2019.
2. UNICEF. End trafficking campaign. 2017. Available at: https://www.unicefusa.org/stories/infographic-global-human-trafficking-statistics. Accessed August 1, 2019.
3. Human Trafficking. The United States Department of Justice website. Available at: https://www.justice.gov/humantrafficking. Accessed July 13, 2019.
4. Smolenski C, Ingerman S. Trafficking of children within the United States. In: Chisolm-Stracker M, Stoklosa H, editors. Human trafficking is a public health issue: a paradigm expansion in the United States. 1st edition. Cham (Switzerland): Springer International Publishing AG; 2017. p. 93–104.
5. Freedom Network USA. Child trafficking for labor in the United States. April 2015. Available at: www.freedomnetworkusa.org/app/uploads/2016/12/HT-and-Child-Labor.pdf. Accessed July 26, 2019.
6. Corbett A. The voices of survivors: an exploration of the contributing factors that assisted with exiting for commercial sexual exploitation in childhood. Child Youth Serv Rev 2017;85:91–8.
7. Greenbaum J, Crawford-Jakubiak J, Committee on Child Abuse and Neglect. Child sex and commercial sexual exploitation: healthcare needs of victims. Pediatrics 2015;135(3):566–74.
8. Gibbs D, Hardison Walters JL, Lutnick A, et al. Evaluation of services for domestic minor victims of human trafficking. Prepared for the U.S. Department of Justice. Research Triangle Park (NC): RTI International; 2014.
9. Clawson HJ, Dutch N, Solomon A, et al. Human trafficking into and within the United States: a review of the literature. Washington, DC: U.S. Department of Health and Human Services, Office of the Assistant Secretary for Planning and Evaluation; 2008.
10. Farrell A, McDevitt J, Fahy S. Understanding and improving law enforcement responses to human trafficking: final report. Washington, DC: Northeastern University Institute on Race and Justice; 2008.

11. Hewetson Gouty A. The best interests of a trafficked adolescent. Ind J Global Legal Stud 2015;22(2):737–67.

12. Farrell A, McDevitt J, Pfeffer R, et al. Identifying challenges to improve the investigation and prosecution of state and local human trafficking cases. 2012. Available at: https://humantraffickinghotline.org/sites/default/files/identifying%20 Challenges%20to%20Prosecution.pdf. Accessed July 29, 2019.

13. Health and healthcare. In: Clayton EW, Krugman RD, Simon P, editors. Confronting commercial sexual exploitation and sex trafficking of minors in the United States. Institute of Medicine and National Research Council of the National Academy. Washington, DC: The National Academies Press; 2013. p. 271–96.

14. National Human Trafficking Hotline website. Hotline statistics. 2018. Available at: https://humantraffickinghotline.org/sites/default/files/2017NHTHStats%20%281% 29.pdf. Accessed July 13, 2019.

15. U.S. Department of Justice. Attorney General's annual report to congress and assessment of U.S. government activities to combat trafficking in person's fiscal year 2017. Available at: https://www.justice.gov/humantrafficking/attorney-generals-trafficking-persons-report. Accessed July 22, 2019.

16. OJJDP. Child labor trafficking. Literature review: a product of the model programs guide 2016. Available at: https://www.ojjdp.gov/mpg/litreviews/child-labor-trafficking.pdf. Accessed August 1, 2019.

17. U.S. State Department. Trafficking in persons report. 2016. Available at: https://www.state.gov/documents/organization/258876.pdf. Accessed July 22, 2019.

18. Wiley KK, Bush K, Scott T. I spy human trafficking? Experts call for mandatory training to identify hidden crimes. ENA Connect 2017;41:15–162.

19. Kenny MC, Helpingstine C, Long H, et al. Increasing child serving professionals' awareness and understanding of the commercial sexual exploitation of children. J Child Sex Abus 2019;28(4):417–34.

20. Sahl S, Knoepke C. Using shared decision making to empower sexually exploited youth. J Am Acad Child Psychiatry 2019;57(11):810–2.

21. Doychak K, Raghavan C. "No voice or vote:" Trauma-coerced attachment in victims of sex trafficking. J Hum Traffick 2018;1–19.

22. Barnert E, Kelly M, Godoy S, et al. Understanding commercially sexually exploited young women's access to, utilization of, and engagement in health care: "work around what I need". Womens Health Issues 2019;29(4):1–10.

23. Roby JL, Vincent M. Federal and state responses to domestic minor sex trafficking: the evolution of policy. Soc Work 2017;62(3):201–9.

24. National Center for Missing and Exploited Children (NCMEC) web page. Available at: http://www.missingkids.com/theissues/trafficking. Accessed July 31, 2019.

25. Polaris. On-ramps, intersections, and exit routes: A roadmap for systems and industries to prevent and disrupt human trafficking. 2018. Available at: https://polarisproject.org/a-roadmap-for-systems-and-industries-to-prevent-and-disrupt-human-trafficking. Accessed November 17, 2019.

26. Beck ME, Lineer MM, Melzer-Lange M, et al. Medical providers' understanding of sex trafficking and their experience with at-risk patients. Pediatrics 2015; 135(4):896.

27. Rajaram S, Tidball S. Survivors' voices: complex needs of sex trafficking survivors in the Midwest. Behav Med 2018;44(3):189–98.

28. Isaac R, Solak J, Giardino A. Health care providers' training needs related to human trafficking: maximizing the opportunity to effectively screen and intervene.

Journ App Research on Children: Informing Policy for Children at Risk 2011; 2(1):8.

29. Dignity Health, HEAL Trafficking, Pacific Survivor Center. PEARR Tool: trauma-informed approach to victim assistance in health care settings; 2019.

30. Alpert EJ, Ahn R, Albright E, et al. Human trafficking: guidebook on identification, assessment, and response in the health care setting. Waltham (MA): MGH Human Trafficking Initiative, Division of Global Health and Human Rights, Department of Emergency Medicine, Massachusetts General Hospital, Boston, MA and Committee on Violence Intervention and Prevention, Massachusetts Medical Society; 2014.

31. Greenbaum VJ, Livings MS, Lai BS, et al. Evaluation of a tool to identify child sex trafficking victims in multiple healthcare settings. J Adolesc Health 2018;63(6): 745–52.

32. National Institute of Justice. A screening tool for identifying trafficking victims. 2016. Available at: https://nij.gov/topics/crime/human-trafficking/Pages/screening-tool-for-identifying-human-trafficking-vicitms.aspx. Accessed July 31, 2019.

Racial Bias and Its Impact on Children and Adolescents

Tiffani J. Johnson, MD, MSc

KEYWORDS

- Bias • Implicit bias • Racism

KEY POINTS

- Similar to the general population, health care providers have implicit racial bias favoring whites. This bias can impact communication and medical decision making, contributing to health care disparities.
- Children and adolescents also experience racial bias in other settings, including the education and criminal justice setting.
- Experiences of bias and discrimination in both health care and general society can have negative impacts on youth academic, behavioral, emotional, and physical health outcomes.
- Research suggests that implicit biases are not hard wired, but can be replaced with new associations with deliberate effort. Health care providers should reflect on their personal attitudes and assumptions, and explore evidence-informed strategies aimed at reducing implicit bias.

INTRODUCTION

As our country continues to become more diverse, pediatricians must be equipped to deliver equitable care to children from different racial and ethnic backgrounds. However, racial and ethnic disparities are pervasive in pediatric health care, with well-documented inequities in child and adolescent mortality, organ transplantation, and quality of care.[1] Although the root causes of such disparities are multifactorial, bias experienced in the health care system and in general society plays an important role.[2] Beyond the immediate psychological impact of bias and discrimination, a life course perspective acknowledges how early childhood experiences of social disadvantage can trigger physiologic responses with cumulative impacts that shape health across an entire life span and across generations.[3]

This article provides a state-of-the-science overview of the impact of racial bias on the health and well-being of children and adolescents. It begins by reviewing the literature on implicit racial bias in health care, with a focus on pediatrics. It then further illustrates youth experience of racial bias in the education and criminal justice setting.

Emergency Medicine, 4150 V Street, Suite 2100, Sacramento, CA 95817, USA
E-mail address: tjo@ucdavis.edu

Pediatr Clin N Am 67 (2020) 425–436
https://doi.org/10.1016/j.pcl.2019.12.011
pediatric.theclinics.com

The article then explores bias as it relates to the broader context of structural racism in America. Next, it provides evidence of the impact of bias and discrimination on youth academic, behavioral, and health outcomes. The article concludes with suggested strategies for confronting implicit bias, addressing structural racism, and promoting the positive development of children from diverse backgrounds. Although this article has focused on racial bias, it is important to acknowledge that other vulnerable and marginalized groups experience bias in society based on socioeconomic status, nationality, language, sex, gender identity, sexual orientation, religion, geography, and disability, as well as the intersectionality of all these diverse populations. These areas warrant further research, particularly as it relates to pediatric patient populations.

RACIAL BIAS IN THE HEALTH CARE SETTING

The landmark Institute of Medicine (now National Academy of Sciences) report "Unequal Treatment," concluded that bias, stereotyping, prejudice, and clinical uncertainty on the part of health care providers may contribute to health care disparities.[2] There is now increasing evidence in the literature confirming the presence of such bias in health care. For example, in a study of medical students and residents, half reported at least one false belief about biological differences between black and white individuals.[4] This included beliefs that black individuals have less sensitive nerve endings, thicker skin, and strong bones in comparison to their white counterparts. These false beliefs were also associated with rating black patients' pain as lower and making less appropriate treatment recommendations.

Beyond explicit beliefs about black patients that providers can self-report, there is a growing body of literature documenting the presence of implicit bias in health care. Implicit bias refers to the attitudes one holds that lie below the surface of one's consciousness, but nevertheless can influence behavior. One way that it can be measured is using the implicit association test (IAT).[5,6] The IAT is a timed categorization task in which participants pair words with faces or names and measures strengths of association using response latency and frequency of errors (https://implicit.harvard.edu/implicit/). The IAT has been used in hundreds of studies across multiple disciplines, with evidence demonstrating that implicit bias is pervasive and impacts behaviors.[7,8]

In addition to research demonstrating that implicit bias is ubiquitous in general society, there is growing evidence that health care providers have similar implicit attitudes favoring white over black and Hispanic patients.[9] Most studies have measured implicit bias using the Adult Race IAT (**Fig. 1**); however, there is also evidence of implicit racial bias toward children in general society, as well as among health care providers using the Child Race IAT (**Fig. 2**). Among nearly 30,000 people who accessed the Child Race IAT on the publicly available Project Implicit Web site, there

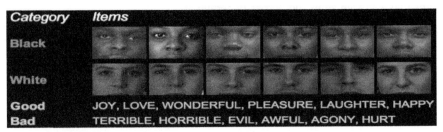

Fig. 1. Stimuli for the Adult Race IAT. This is a timed task in which participants categorize pictures of black and white adult faces and words that represent the constructs of good and bad.

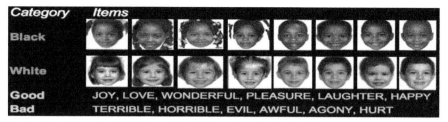

Category	Items
Black	
White	
Good	JOY, LOVE, WONDERFUL, PLEASURE, LAUGHTER, HAPPY
Bad	TERRIBLE, HORRIBLE, EVIL, AWFUL, AGONY, HURT

Fig. 2. Stimuli for the Child Race IAT. This is a timed task in which participants categorize pictures of black and white children's faces and words that represent the constructs of good and bad.

was implicit pro-white/anti-black bias toward children similar to levels of bias found on the Adult Race IAT.[10] Research using the Child Race IAT among child and adult participants has also found implicit bias favoring white children over black children.[11,12]

Two studies, both in the emergency department setting, have measured implicit racial bias toward children among physicians.[13,14] One found that most resident physicians working in a pediatric emergency department had IAT scores consistent with pro-white/anti-black racial bias on both the Adult Race IAT (85%) and Child Race IAT (91%).[13] There were no significant differences in levels of bias toward adults versus children, and bias did not vary based on resident demographic characteristics, including gender and specialty when comparing pediatric resident physicians with emergency medicine residents. In another study of emergency department providers at 5 hospitals in the Midwest, 84% had implicit bias in favor of white children in comparison with American Indian children.[14] This study also found that explicit attitudes varied by practice setting, with American Indian children being perceived as increasingly challenging and their parents as less compliant as the proportion of American Indians seen at the site increased. These studies suggest that, similar to adult patients, children are also vulnerable to biased racial attitudes from their health care providers.

Although we know bias impacts decisions in other sectors of society, studies examining the impact that provider bias has on medical decision making have mixed results and largely focus on adult populations using clinical vignettes.[9] For example, physician implicit bias has been linked with disparities in treatment recommendations for adults with chest pain and type II diabetes mellitus.[15,16] In contrast, other studies using clinical vignettes found no association between implicit bias and medical decision making in the areas of adult trauma care,[17–20] osteosteoarthritis,[21] or pain management.[18,22]

Other research has demonstrated that racial bias was associated with differences in assessment of case vignettes depicting black and white patients with chest pain only when time pressure was experimentally induced.[23] This is important, considering the time pressure that health care providers face in both the acute and primary care settings. Additional evidence shows that cognitive stressors such as emergency department overcrowding and caring for more patients during a shift is associated with increased implicit bias.[13] Beyond the day-to-day pressures of clinical care impacting racial bias, providers' attitudes are also impacted by chronic stress and burnout. In a study of resident physicians, self-reported symptoms of burnout, in particular, depersonalization, were associated with more unfavorable attitudes toward black people, with greater levels of both explicit and implicit bias.[24]

Fewer studies have investigated the impact of implicit bias on medical decision making in pediatrics. A vignette study looking at bias toward American Indian children found no association between measures of implicit or explicit bias and medical decision making.[14] However, another study revealed that pediatric providers with greater implicit pro-white/anti-black bias were more likely to prescribe narcotic medications for postsurgical pain for white patients and more likely to disagree with prescribing narcotics for black patients with postsurgical pain.[25]

When examining the impact of bias on real world patient outcomes, investigators found that adult patients with spinal cord injuries had worse social integration, depression, and life satisfaction if their physician had more implicit racial bias.[26] However, another study found no association between implicit provider bias and hypertension treatment decisions, patient adherence, or blood pressure control.[27] It should be noted that the patients in this study received regular care from the same health care provider for an average of 9 visits across 3 years. This may suggest that building trusting therapeutic patient-provider relationships over time, in conjunction with clear evidence-based guidelines, may help buffer the impact of bias on patient care. Additional research is needed to further explore the impact of racial biases on real world pediatric patient care.

In addition to its potential impact on medical decision making, bias also can impact how providers communicate with patients. There is consistent and robust evidence that physicians with higher implicit bias demonstrate higher verbal dominance in their communication styles, less interpersonal treatment, less supportive communication, and less patient-centered communication.[28–34] Furthermore, the patients of providers with higher implicit bias report poorer ratings of satisfaction, and greater difficulty with following recommendations.[34] There is also evidence suggesting that provider bias impacts communication with pediatric patients. A study examining recorded interviews of acute care office visits found that pediatricians were less likely to ask black children to answer questions than white children, independent of the child's age.[35] Additional research is needed in the pediatric health care setting to further explore the impact of provider bias on communication with patients and their families and how this impacts therapeutic bonds, satisfaction, and adherence with treatment recommendations.

BIAS IN THE EDUCATION AND JUSTICE SETTING

In addition to experiences in health care, children and adolescents also experienced bias and discrimination in the educational setting that can have negative impacts on their well-being. For example, in a study in which educators were asked to look for deviant behaviors when shown video clips of children engaging in typical activities, eye trackers revealed longer gazes at black children compared with white children, which was most pronounced for black male children.[36] These biases in expectations for misbehavior may explain why children of color, especially black boys, face higher rates of suspension and expulsion from kindergarten.[37]

Bias may also lead to devaluation of students based on implicitly or explicitly held beliefs, resulting in educators being dismissive of students' aspirations. For example, minority high school students report receiving lower grades than deserved, being unfairly disciplined based on race, and being discouraged from joining an advanced-level class.[38] These perceptions are supported by data indicating that 75% of Native American students, 72% of black students, and 66% of Hispanic students whose standardized testing scores suggested they had the potential to be successful in advanced-placement math, were not enrolled in those advanced classes. There were similar findings for advanced-placement science classes.[39] Research also shows that the implicit pro-white bias of instructors is predictive of lower test scores for their black learners. This relationship was mediated by instructors' anxiety and poor lesson quality.[40] Teachers also direct less praise, affirmations, and questions toward black and Latino students compared with white students.[41] The impact of these experiences of bias in education on youth can include poor school engagement as well as poor academic motivation.[42,43]

The pervasiveness of bias toward youth also extends to the justice system. For example, black and Hispanic sexual abuse victims are perceived as being more responsible for their abuse in comparison with white victims.[44] Black and Latino boys in the juvenile justice system are perceived as being older than their actual age and more culpable for their crimes in comparison with their white peers.[45] Furthermore, a study in which police officers were given an implicit dehumanization task found that the more officers implicitly associated blacks with apes, the more frequently they had used force against black children relative to children of other races throughout their careers.[45]

STRUCTURAL RACISM

It is important for health care provides to acknowledge and address biases experienced by children and adolescents in health care and general society. Even when implicit and unintentional, bias represents a form of personally mediated racism that negatively impacts youth. It is also important for health care providers to recognize the broader existence of structural racism in America. Structural racism operationalizes itself though policies, laws, and regulations on a local, state, and national level that results in differential access to the goods, services, and opportunities based on race.[46] One example of structural racism is redlining, or marking neighborhoods based on racial demographics as hazardous in red ink on maps drawn by the federal Home Owners' Loan Corp in the 1930s.[47] Redlining led to the systematic denial of capital investments that could improve the house and economic opportunities of residents, leading to subsequent impact on services such as health care, supermarkets, and transportation. The legacy of redlining has persistent impacts on children, as 74% of neighborhoods redlined as hazardous 80 years ago are low to moderate income today, and 64% are minority neighborhoods today.[47] This resulting residential segregation has many impacts on where children live, learn, and play; including access to safe playgrounds, grocery stores with nutritious foods, public transportation, and quality schools. In the education setting, for example, allocation of resources across lines of race and class leads to inequities in the quality and experience of teachers and the quality and rigor of the curriculum.[48] Another example of how racism also operationalizes itself at the structural level is through disciplinary policies and practices in schools that lead to criminalizing youth behaviors, increasing their contact with law enforcement, and funneling them into the criminal justice system, often referred to as the school to prison pipeline.[49]

IMPACT OF RACISM AND BIAS ON HEALTH AND WELL-BEING

Whether it exists on the implicit, explicit, or structural level, racism has important impacts on the health and well-being of children and adolescents. A robust body of literature has shown a strong and consistent relationship between general self-reported experiences of racial bias and discrimination with poor emotional outcomes, including emotional distress, depressive symptoms, stress, anxiety, general self-efficacy, and feelings of hopelessness and powerlessness.[43,50–53] Researchers have also identified experiences of racism as a robust predictor of delinquent behaviors, including acts of violence and aggression.[54–56] It is also important for pediatric providers to recognize that youth who face the daily barrage of structural and personally mediated racism in their lives may then accept negative messages about their own abilities and self-worth. This internalized racism may be manifested as poor school performance, high drop-out rates, and engagement in high-risk behaviors that can have negative impacts on health. Internalized racism has been linked with increased metabolic health risk in adolescent girls, including insulin resistance and larger waist circumference.[57] The toxic stress of experiencing racial bias and discrimination also can trigger physiologic responses that increase risk for chronic disease across the life course and result in overall poor self-reported health status and disparities in health outcomes, including elevated blood pressure, heart disease, diabetes, and low infant birth rate.[52,58–61]

EVIDENCE-BASED STRATEGIES FOR REDUCING IMPLICIT BIAS

Acknowledging that bias plays a role in the care delivered, pediatric providers have an opportunity to examine their own biases and consider how they may influence clinical practice. Efforts to incorporate awareness of implicit bias in medical school and residency training programs are important steps in training the next generation of pediatricians to treat patients and families with respect and provide high-quality care to an increasingly diverse patient population. There remains a need to help practicing providers beyond training, particularly those in leadership roles, confront their personal biases and mitigate their impact on patient care, and medical and graduate medical education, as well as the recruitment and advancement of a diverse pediatric workforce.

Although there is a dearth of evidence-based interventions to reduce bias in health care, practitioners can turn to strategies found to be successful in other settings. Perspective taking, whereby individuals consciously assess a situation from the point of another racial group, is one example of a strategy that has shown success for both implicit and explicit tasks.[62] This could be applied to pediatric health care by considering the experiences, feelings, and thinking of patients and families from different backgrounds as a strategy to build empathy and understanding. This can include reflecting on what barriers they face when trying to access the health care system (eg, insurance, transportation, other familial and work obligations), and considering how their past experiences in society and the health care system may influence their attitudes, behaviors, and communication style. Research also shows that exploring common identities can reduce in-group versus out-group thinking and implicit bias.[63] This can help individuals focus on the things held in common with people from different backgrounds instead of just focusing on cultural, social, and demographic differences. There is also a growing body of evidence showing that mindfulness interventions are effective at reducing implicit bias.[64–67] Mindfulness-based practices also can offer other benefits to health care providers, including decreasing burnout and improving empathy and well-being.[68,69] In another successful intervention, after completing a baseline IAT and an educational program about the impact of implicit bias on discriminatory behaviors, participants were trained on how to apply several bias-reduction strategies to everyday life. These strategies included (1) *stereotype replacement*, where individuals were trained to recognize stereotypes being perpetuated in society and within themselves and how to replace them with non-stereotypic responses; (2) *counter-stereotypic imaging*, imagining someone from a marginalized group who does not fulfill commonly believed stereotypes about that group; (3) *individuation*, where one tries to get to know someone else and focus on their individual characteristics instead of their group-based characteristics, which can often be influenced by stereotypes; (4) *perspective taking*; and (5) *increasing opportunity for cross-cultural contact*.[70]

Despite the promising results from these other studies, research aimed at reducing implicit bias in the health care setting is limited. One study found that a multicultural training course reduced implicit bias by 9% when compared with controls.[71] In a pilot study among 69 pediatric resident trainees, a 2-part facilitated group intervention using photodocumentaries found increased empathy and patient centeredness in the intervention compared with a control group. White participants in the intervention group also demonstrated decreased implicit biases toward Latino individuals regarding pleasantness.[72] In a study among medical students, a health equity curriculum was found to reduce implicit biases regarding sexuality and race. The curriculum included taking an IAT; a debriefing session; and a 2-hour session that focused on enhancing internal motivation to reduce bias, understanding the psychological basis of bias, increasing participants' confidence in their ability to successfully interact with patients from different social backgrounds, emotional regulation skills, and building partnerships with patients.[73] Additional research is needed to further investigate how these bias-reduction strategies impact the delivery of more equitable patient care and more effective cross-cultural communication.

Additional insight can be gained from research exploring how provider implicit bias changes over time. For example, a study looking at medical students' changes in implicit racial bias over the course of their medical education found increased bias associated with hearing negative comments about minority patients from faculty members, whereas favorable contact with black faculty members was associated with reduced bias.[74] Research on how clinical workday factors impact bias suggests that addressing factors that can contribute to cognitive stress in the clinical environment, such as patient overcrowding, interruptions when performing clinical tasks, and time pressure, as well as the use of evidence-based decision support tools to decrease cognitive load, may reduce the impact of bias on clinical decision making.[13] Strategies to reduce burnout also are needed to improve empathy and reduce the impact of bias on patient care. Research suggests that such interventions should be organization-directed, as opposed to individual-directed.[75,76]

THE ROLE OF HEALTH CARE IN ADDRESSING STRUCTURAL RACISM

Although it is important to acknowledge and address personal biases to achieve excellence in the care of children and adolescents, pediatric providers also need to be active champions of antiracism through clinical practice, advocacy, and research. This requires acknowledging past and present policies that fuel social determinants of health, and engaging in partnerships with patients, families, community members, and policymakers to play a meaningful role in developing solutions to address these social determinants. In clinical practice, this can begin with identifying and addressing the systems, policies, and procedures in place in clinics and hospitals that can perpetuate inequities. Providers also must be prepared to have critical and developmentally appropriate conversations with patients and families about racism. In a policy statement on the impact of racism on child and adolescent health, the American Academy of Pediatrics offers several strategies for optimizing anticipatory guidance around this topic, such as racial socialization to help combat internalized racism.[77] Beyond the role of individual providers, youth-serving organizations also must make racial equity a strategic priority and can help dismantle structural racism by serving as anchor institutions, investing in the community to promote health, and supporting economic vitality.[78,79]

SUMMARY

Racial bias is pervasive throughout society and can impact children and adolescents in the health care, education, and criminal justice system. Not only can provider bias have impacts on patient care and communication, but experiences of bias and discrimination have impacts on health outcomes across the life course. It is important for pediatricians to identify and confront their own personal biases, support equity within the structure of the health care system, and advocate more broadly for policies that help dismantle structural racism.

DISCLOSURE

None.

REFERENCES

1. Flores G. Technical report–racial and ethnic disparities in the health and health care of children. Pediatrics 2010;125(4):e979–1020.
2. Smedley B, Stith AY, Nelson A, editors. Unequal treatment: confronting racial and ethnic disparities in health care. Washington, DC: National Academies Press; 2002.
3. Jones NL, Gilman SE, Cheng TL, et al. Life course approaches to the causes of health disparities. Am J Public Health 2019;109(S1):S48–55.
4. Hoffman KM, Trawalter S, Axt JR, et al. Racial bias in pain assessment and treatment recommendations, and false beliefs about biological differences between blacks and whites. Proc Natl Acad Sci U S A 2016;113(16):4296–301.
5. Greenwald AG, McGhee DE, Schwartz JL. Measuring individual differences in implicit cognition: the implicit association test. J Pers Soc Psychol 1998;74(6):1464–80.
6. Greenwald AG, Nosek BA, Banaji MR. Understanding and using the implicit association test: I. An improved scoring algorithm. J Pers Soc Psychol 2003;85(2):197–216.
7. Nosek BA, Greenwald AG, Banaji MR. The implicit association test at age 7: a methodological and conceptual review. In: Bargh JA, editor. Automatic processes in social thinking and behavior. Psychology Press; 2007. p. 265–92.
8. Dasgupta N. Implicit ingroup favoritism, outgroup favoritism, and their behavioral manifestations. Soc Justice Res 2004;17:143–69.
9. Maina IW, Belton TD, Ginzberg S, et al. A decade of studying implicit racial/ethnic bias in healthcare providers using the implicit association test. Soc Sci Med 2018;199:219–29.
10. Lane KA, Banaji MR, Nosek BA, et al. Understanding and using the Implicit Association Test. IV. What we know (so far) about the method. In: Wittenbrink B, Schwarz N, editors. Implicit measures of attitudes. New York: Guilford Press; 2007. p. 59–102.
11. Baron AS, Banaji MR. The development of implicit attitudes. Evidence of race evaluations from ages 6 and 10 and adulthood. Psychol Sci 2006;17:53–8.
12. Newheiser AK, Olson KR. White and black American children's implicit intergroup bias. J Exp Soc Psychol 2012;48:264–70.
13. Johnson TJ, Hickey RW, Switzer GE, et al. The impact of cognitive stressors in the emergency department on physician implicit racial bias. Acad Emerg Med 2016;23(3):297–305.

14. Puumala SE, Burgess KM, Kharbanda AB, et al. The role of bias by emergency department providers in care for American Indian children. Med Care 2016; 54(6):562–9.
15. Green AR, Carney DR, Pallin DJ, et al. Implicit bias among physicians and its prediction of thrombolysis decisions for black and white patients. J Gen Intern Med 2007;22(9):1231–8.
16. Charles L. Causal and predictive relationships among race, implicit racial bias, and simulated treatment recommendations. Available from ProWuest Dissertations & theses Global: the sciences and Engineering Collection. 2009.
17. Haider AH, Schneider EB, Sriram N, et al. Unconscious race and social class bias among acute care surgical clinicians and clinical treatment decisions. JAMA Surg 2015;150(5):457–64.
18. Haider AH, Sexton J, Sriram N, et al. Association of unconscious race and social class bias with vignette-based clinical assessments by medical students. JAMA 2011;306(9):942–51.
19. Haider AH, Schneider EB, Sriram N, et al. Unconscious race and class biases among registered nurses: vignette-based study using implicit association testing. J Am Coll Surg 2015;220(6):1077–86.e3.
20. Haider AH, Schneider EB, Sriram N, et al. Unconscious race and class bias: its association with decision making by trauma and acute care surgeons. J Trauma Acute Care Surg 2014;77(3):409–16.
21. Oliver MN, Wells KM, Joy-Gaba JA, et al. Do physicians' implicit views of African Americans affect clinical decision making? J Am Board Fam Med 2014;27(2): 177–88.
22. Hirsh AT, Hollingshead NA, Ashburn-Nardo L, et al. The interaction of patient race, provider bias, and clinical ambiguity on pain management decisions. J Pain 2015;16(6):558–68.
23. Stepanikova I. Racial-ethnic biases, time pressure, and medical decisions. J Health Soc Behav 2012;53:329–43.
24. Dyrbye L, Herrin J, West CP, et al. Association of racial bias with burnout among resident physicians. JAMA Netw Open 2019;2(7):e197457.
25. Sabin JA, Greenwald AG. The influence of implicit bias on treatment recommendations for 4 common pediatric conditions: pain, urinary tract infection, attention deficit hyperactivity disorder, and asthma. Am J Public Health 2012;102(5): 988–95.
26. Hausmann LR, Myaskovsky L, Niyonkuru C, et al. Examining implicit bias of physicians who care for individuals with spinal cord injury: a pilot study and future directions. J Spinal Cord Med 2015;38(1):102–10.
27. Blair IV, Steiner JF, Hanratty R, et al. An investigation of associations between clinicians' ethnic or racial bias and hypertension treatment, medication adherence and blood pressure control. J Gen Intern Med 2014;29(7):987–95.
28. Cooper LA, Roter DL, Carson KA, et al. The associations of clinicians' implicit attitudes about race with medical visit communication and patient ratings of interpersonal care. Am J Public Health 2012;102(5):979–87.
29. Blair IV, Steiner JF, Fairclough DL, et al. Clinicians' implicit ethnic/racial bias and perceptions of care among Black and Latino patients. Ann Fam Med 2013;11(1): 43–52.
30. Hagiwara N, Penner LA, Gonzalez R, et al. Racial attitudes, physician-patient talk time ratio, and adherence in racially discordant medical interactions. Soc Sci Med 2013;87:123–31.

31. Hagiwara N, Slatcher RB, Eggly S, et al. Physician racial bias and word use during racially discordant medical interactions. Health Commun 2016;32(4):1–8.

32. Hagiwara N, Dovidio JF, Eggly S, et al. The effects of racial attitudes on affect and engagement in racially discordant medical interactions between non-Black physicians and Black patients. Group Process Intergroup Relat 2016;19(4):509–27.

33. Penner LA, Dovidio JF, West TV, et al. Aversive racism and medical interactions with black patients: a field study. J Exp Soc Psychol 2010;46(2):436–40.

34. Penner LA, Dovidio JF, Gonzalez R, et al. The effects of oncologist implicit racial bias in racially discordant oncology interactions. J Clin Oncol 2016;34(24):2874–80.

35. Stivers T, Majid A. Questioning children: interactional evidence of implicit bias in medical interviews. Soc Psychol Q 2007;70:424–41.

36. Gilliam W, Maupin A, Reyes C, et al. Do early educators' implicit biases regarding sex and race relate to behavior expectations and recommendations of preschool expulsions and suspensions? New Haven (CT): Yale Child Study Center; 2016. Available at: http://ziglercenter.yale.edu/publications/Preschool%20Implicit%20Bias%20Policy%20Brief_final_9_26_276766_5379.pdf.

37. US Department of Education. Data snapshot: early childhood education. Washington, DC: Civil Rights Data Collection; 2014. p. 1–17.

38. Fisher C, Wallace S, Fenton R. Discrimination distress during adolescence. J Youth Adolesc 2000;29(6):679–95.

39. Theokas C, Saaris R. Finding America's missing AP and IB students. shattering expectations series. Washington, DC: The Education Trust; 2013. Available at: https://edtrust.org/wp-content/uploads/2013/10/Missing_Students.pdf.

40. Jacoby-Senghor DS, Sinclair S, Shelton JN. A lesson in bias: the relationship between implicit racial bias and performance in pedagogical contexts. J Exp Soc Psychol 2016;63:50–5.

41. Tenenbaum HR, Ruck MD. Are teachers' expectations different for racial minority than for European American students? A meta-analysis. J Educ Psychol 2007;99(2):253–73.

42. Dotterer AM, McHale SM, Crouter AC. Sociocultural factors and school engagement among African American youth: the roles of racial discrimination, racial socialization and ethnic identity. Appl Dev Sci 2009;13(2):51–73.

43. Wong CA, Eccles JS, Sameroff A. The influence of ethnic discrimination and ethnic identification on African American adolescents' school and socioemotional adjustment. J Pers 2003;71(6):1197–232.

44. Bottoms BL, Davis SL. Effect of victim and defendant race on jurors' decisions in child sex abuse cases. J Appl Soc Psychol 2004;34(1):1–33.

45. Goff PA, Jackson MC, Di Leone BA, et al. The essence of innocence: consequences of dehumanizing Black children. J Pers Soc Psychol 2014;106(4):526–45.

46. Jones C. Confronting institutionalized racism. Phylon 2003;50(1–2):7–22.

47. Mitchell B, Franco J. HOLC "redlining" maps: the persistent structure of segregation and economic inequality. Washington, DC: National Community Reinvestment Coalition; 2018. Available at: https://ncrc.org/holc/.

48. US Commission on Civil Rights. Public education funding inequity in an era of increasing concentration of poverty and resegregation. Washington, DC: 2018. Available at: https://www.usccr.gov/pubs/2018/2018-01-10-Education-Inequity.pdf. Accessed April 19, 2019.

49. Wald J, Losen DJ. Defining and redirecting a school-to-prison pipeline. New Dir Youth Dev 2003;99:9–15.

50. Simons R, Murry V, McLoyd V, et al. Discrimination, crime, ethnic identity, and parenting as correlates of depressive symptoms among African American children: a multilevel analysis. Dev Psychopathol 2002;14(2):371–93.

51. Scott LD Jr. Correlates of coping with perceived discriminatory experiences among African American adolescents. J Adolesc 2004;27(2):123–37.

52. Paradies Y. A systematic review of empirical research on self-reported racism and health. Int J Epidemiol 2006;35(4):888–901.

53. Gibbons FX, Yeh HC, Gerrard M, et al. Early experience with racial discrimination and conduct disorder as predictors of subsequent drug use: a critical period hypothesis. Drug Alcohol Depend 2007;88(Suppl 1):S2737.

54. Simons R, Chen Y, Stewart E, et al. Incidence of discrimination and risk for delinquency: a longitudinal test of strain theory with an African American sample. Justice Q 2003;20(4):827–54.

55. Caldwell C, Kohn-Wood L, Schmeelk-Cone K, et al. Racial discrimination and racial identity as risk or protective factors for violent behaviors in African American young adults. Am J Community Psychol 2004;33(1–2):91–105.

56. Burt CH, Simons RL, Gibbons FX. Racial discrimination, ethnic-racial socialization, and crime: a micro-sociological model of risk and resilience. Am Sociol Rev 2012;77(4):648–77.

57. Chambers EC, Tull ES, Fraser HS, et al. The relationship of internalized racism to body fat distribution and insulin resistance among African adolescent youth. J Natl Med Assoc 2004;96(12):1594–8.

58. Clark R, Anderson NB, Clark VR, et al. Racism as a stressor for African Americans. A biopsychosocial model. Am Psychol 1999;54(10):805–16.

59. Mays VM, Cochran SD, Barnes NW. Race, race-based discrimination, and health outcomes among African Americans. Annu Rev Psychol 2007;58:201–25.

60. Schulz A, Israel B, Williams D, et al. Social inequalities, stressors and self reported health status among African American and white women in the Detroit metropolitan area. Soc Sci Med 2000;51(11):1639–53.

61. Gee GC, Walsemann KM, Brandolo E. A life course perspective on how racism may be related to health disparities. Am J Public Health 2012;102(5):967–74.

62. Galinsky AD, Moskowitz GB. Perspective-taking: decreasing stereotype expression, stereotype accessibility, and in-group favoritism. J Pers Soc Psychol 2000; 78(4):708–24.

63. Hall NR, Crisp RJ. Reducing implicit prejudice by blurring intergroup boundaries. Basic Appl Soc Psychol 2009;31(3):244–54.

64. Lueke A, Gibson B. Brief mindfulness meditation reduces discrimination. Psychology of Consciousness: Theory, Research, and Practice 2016;3(1):34–44.

65. Kang Y, Gray JR, Dovidio JF. The nondiscriminating heart: loving kindness meditation training decreases implicit intergroup bias. J Exp Psychol Gen 2014; 143(3):1306–13.

66. Stell AJ, Farsides T. Brief loving-kindness meditation reduces racial bias, mediated by positive other-regarding emotions. Motiv Emot 2015;40:140–7.

67. Parks S, Birtel MD, Crisp RJ. Evidence that a brief meditation exercise can reduce prejudice toward homeless people. Soc Psychol 2014;45(6):458–65.

68. Goodman MJ, Schorling JB. A mindfulness course decreases burnout and improved well-being among healthcare providers. Int J Psychiatry Med 2012; 43(2):119–28.

69. Krasner MS, Epstein RM, Beckman H, et al. Association of an educational program in mindful communication with burnout, empathy and attitudes among primary care physicians. JAMA 2009;302(12):1284–93.

70. Devine PG, Forscher PS, Austin AJ, et al. Long-term reduction in implicit race bias: a prejudice habit-breaking intervention. J Exp Soc Psychol 2012;48(6): 1267–78.

71. Castillo L, Reyes C, Brossart D, et al. The influence of multicultural training on perceived multicultural counseling competencies and implicit racial prejudice. J Multicult Counsel Dev 2007;35(4):243–54.

72. Chapman MV, Hall WJ, Lee K, et al. Making a difference in medical trainees' attitudes towards Latino patients: a pilot study of an intervention to modify implicit and explicit attitudes. Soc Sci Med 2018;199:202–8.

73. Leslie KF, Sawning S, Shaw MA, et al. Changes in medical student implicit attitudes following a health equity curricular intervention. Med Teach 2018;40(4): 372–8.

74. van Ryn M, Hardeman R, Phelan SM, et al. Medical school experiences associated with change in implicit racial bias among 3547 students: a Medical Student CHANGES Study Report. J Gen Intern Med 2015;30(12):1748–56.

75. Panagioti M, Panagopoulou E, Bower P, et al. Controlled interventions to reduce burnout in physicians: a systematic review and meta-analysis. JAMA Intern Med 2017;177(2):195–205.

76. Linzer M, Poplau S, Grossman E, et al. A cluster randomized trial of interventions to improve work conditions and clinician burnout in primary care: results from the Healthy Work Place (HWP) study. J Gen Intern Med 2015;30(8):1105–11.

77. Trent M, Dooley DG, Douge J. The impact of racism on child and adolescent health. Pediatrics 2019;144(2):1–14.

78. Task Force on Anchor Institutions. Anchor institutions as partners in building successful communities and local economies. In: Brophy PC, Godsil RD, editors. Retooling HUD for a catalytic federal government: a report to Secretary Shaun Donovan. Philadelphia: Penn Institute for Urban Research; 2009. p. 147–69. Available at: http://www.margainc.com/initiatives/aitf.

79. Harkavy I. Engaging urban universities as anchor institutions for health equity. Am J Public Health 2016;106(12):2155–7.

Printed and bound by CPI Group (UK) Ltd, Croydon, CR0 4YY

03/10/2024

01040400-0019